CHOOSING HEALTHY MEALS FROM THE FOODS YOU LOVE

Discover all the information you need to stay fit and healthy while dining out on your favorite foods from around the globe. The most practical guide of its kind, it provides all the tools you need to make sensible and delicious dining choices, including:

- Tips for ordering what you want exactly the way you want it prepared

- An overview of popular dishes—which are the best and which are the worst for fat-conscious dieters

- Ingredient lists for all of your favorite ethnic foods

- A "Staples" section which lists common foods and the nutritional contents of dishes not listed in the charts

THE ESSENTIAL FAT GRAM COUNTER FOR ETHNIC DINING

MARISA SIMMS

Produced by The Philip Lief Group, Inc.

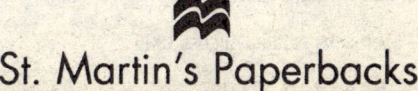

St. Martin's Paperbacks

NOTE: If you purchased this book without a cover you should be aware that this book is stolen property. It was reported as "unsold and destroyed" to the publisher, and neither the author nor the publisher has received any payment for this "stripped book."

When using nutritional analyses for medicinal purposes, the reader should bear in mind that this book is intended to serve as a general reference only, and should not be used to replace the advice of a physician. Responsibility for any adverse effects or unforeseen consequences of the use of information contained in this book is expressly disclaimed by the author and the publisher.

Produced by The Philip Lief Group, Inc.

THE ESSENTIAL FAT GRAM COUNTER FOR ETHNIC DINING

Copyright © 1996 by the Philip Lief Group, Inc.

Cover photograph by Herman Estévez.

All rights reserved. No part of this book may be used or reproduced in any manner whatsoever without written permission except in the case of brief quotations embodied in critical articles or reviews. For information address St. Martin's Press, 175 Fifth Avenue, New York, N.Y. 10010.

ISBN: 0-312-95933-8

Printed in the United States of America

St. Martin's Paperbacks edition/August 1996

10 9 8 7 6 5 4 3 2 1

Contents

INTRODUCTION	1
A Guide to Healthy Eating	5
Common Fats and Oils	8
The Cuisines	11
African	13
Caribbean	21
Chinese	29
French	53
German and Austrian	77
Greek and Middle Eastern	85
Indian	93
Italian	107
Japanese	139
Mexican	151
Russian and Eastern European	179
Spanish	187
Thai	195
Staples	215
Weekly Food Chart	233

Introduction

The Essential Fat Gram Counter for Ethnic Dining is designed to help you make intelligent choices in the menus of different cultures and also to inspire you to ask questions about the food you eat every day. Once you become familiar with—and appreciate—the many ethnic foods that are as delicious as they are healthy, you can eat anywhere with confidence . . . without adding extra pounds.

Health-conscious diners are often at a loss when it comes to ordering from the menu of another cuisine, because many of the ingredients are unfamiliar. Is palm kernel oil good or bad? What's inside a chile relleno (stuffed chile)? Usually ethnic restaurants include helpful descriptions on the menu, but many restaurants dispense with information about ingredients. Also, it is quite common for the menu to be written in the language of the culture. How many of us have struggled with the menu in a French or Italian restaurant? At times like these, ordering can become a question of eenie-meenie-miney-moe—not the best way to choose how much fat is going into your body. This book helps eliminate that guesswork.

Today most physicians and nutritionists recognize that eating less fat is an essential component of a healthy diet. Gram for gram, fat contains more than twice the calories of carbohydrates and protein. Unfortunately, many Americans are accustomed to eating a high-fat, high-cholesterol, high-sodium diet, and statistics show that we are paying the price not only with high incidences of cancer, but with increased rates of high blood pressure, heart attacks, and strokes. A low-fat diet may actually reduce your risk of certain types of cancer, particularly those of the breast, colon, prostate, and uterus.

Some Tricks to Help You Avoid Overeating

Temptation is everywhere and even the most disciplined dieters will occasionally lose their willpower and overfill their plates when faced with an attractive buffet or a fabulous home-cooked meal. There are, however, several little tricks everyone can use when eating out to avoid consuming extra calories and fat:

- One way to avoid overeating is to take the edge off your hunger in the beginning of the meal by starting off with a healthy low-calorie soup, salad, or appetizer. Broth-based soups; raw or steamed vegetables; unbuttered bread, breadsticks, or popcorn; and small seafood appetizers prepared without butter or heavy sauces can help fill you up before your main course arrives. If you are skipping the first course, drink a glass of water or tea just before your meal.
- When choosing entrees, pay close attention to how foods are prepared. This is a surefire way to avoid ingesting hidden calories. Select menu items that are steamed, poached, broiled, roasted, baked, or cooked in their own juices. Avoid foods that are fried, sautéed, breaded, or covered with cheese.
- Lots of calories and extra fat can be eliminated if you simply remove the skin from poultry before eating it; also trim the excess fat from red meat to effect savings.
- Avoid heavy, creamy sauces at all costs! Sauces such as hollandaise, béarnaise, beurre blanc, and most gravies are loaded with fat. Instead choose tomato-based sauces (without cream added), soy-based sauces (unless you are on a low-sodium diet), or sauces that are designated low-fat on the menu.
- If you're unsure about the contents of a sauce or dressing, ask that it be served on the side and use it sparingly. When selecting salad dressing, choose lemon juice, plain vinegar, or yogurt-based ones. In general, it's best to avoid thick dressings like Russian, and creamy dressings like ranch, unless they are special low-fat blends.
- Eat slowly, and stop eating as soon as you feel satisfied. Don't wait until you are so full you need to undo that button! Order half-portions when they are available. After all, as the old adage goes—it's better to waste, than to your waist!

- Skip dessert as a rule, and on those few occasions when dessert looks just too delicious to pass up, limit yourself to just a taste—then share the treat with the rest of your dining companions. Many forks make for fewer calories—and less guilt! Another option is to order fresh fruit, if it is on the menu.

When in Doubt, Ask Your Waiter

Most restaurants and cooks now recognize that diners want to have plenty of healthy options available to them, and are very willing to honor special requests. Don't be shy! If you are truly committed to monitoring your fat intake, on occasion you may need to order something special for yourself that doesn't appear on the menu. If you are eating out, and you're concerned about the fat content of a particular dish, remember that the wait staff are there to help you order exactly what you want, and to make sure you are happy with the way your meal is cooked. Many restaurants offer delicious vegetarian and low-fat dishes. These are often noted as such on the menu. Wherever you are eating, don't be afraid to ask questions and make reasonable requests.

Once you are committed to lowering your fat intake, you will find that there's no better place to start than with food from other cultures. Sensible eating is painless and enjoyable when you treat your tastebuds to new culinary wonders on a regular basis.

A Guide to Healthy Eating

Every dish listed in *The Essential Fat Gram Counter for Ethnic Dining* is followed by a complete nutritional breakdown. When interpreting the analysis that follows each dish, use the informative guidelines below to help you evaluate what you are about to eat.

CALORIES: An individual's ideal daily caloric intake can vary greatly. It's important to take into account factors such as whether you are more or less physically active than the average person, whether you are trying to lose, maintain, or gain weight, and any medical conditions you have that affect your diet, including pregnancy. The best way to be sure you are eating the right amount of calories is to ask your doctor. However, there are some generally accepted guidelines, which can help you determine how many calories a day you should consume:

- Adults can use 1,700 to 3,000 calories a day
- Adolescent boys and very active men under 55 can utilize close to 3,000 calories a day
- Men over the age of 55 need roughly 2,500 calories per day
- Women from their teens to 35 need about 2,000 calories daily
- Very active women need 2,400 calories per day
- Women who are pregnant need 2,200 calories daily, and women who are lactating need 3,000 calories per day
- Women over 55 need only about 1,700 calories per day
- Children from one to six need approximately 1,100 to 1,600 calories per day
- Under the age of one year, a baby's caloric intake needs to be closely monitored and parents should consult with their pediatrician to determine the infant's diet

- In order to meet basic nutritional requirements, it is not advisable for women to eat fewer than 1,200 calories per day; men should not consume fewer than 1,500 calories per day

FAT: The American Heart Association, the American Health Foundation, the American Cancer Society, and the Surgeon General all recommend that no more than 30 percent of your caloric intake be made up of fat, and some experts feel that a diet which contains only 25 percent fat is ideal.

In order to determine how many fat grams you should allow yourself on a daily basis, multiply your daily caloric intake by .3, and divide the total by 9 (there are 9 calories in a gram of fat). For example, a 1,500-calorie-per-day diet would look like this:

1,500 calories $\times$ .3 = 450 / 9 = 50 grams of fat daily

Adults need a minimum daily intake of 15 to 25 grams of fat to meet basic nutritional needs.

You might be surprised to learn that not all fat is bad for you. In fact, some fats are essential for the normal maintenance and development of the body. Fats act as fuel and insulation against cold, as cushioning for the internal organs, and as lubricants. Fats make it possible for us to utilize such fat-soluble vitamins as A, D, E, and K. Fat also helps us manufacture antibodies that fight infections and diseases.

There are two types of fat in our bodies. These are the nonessential fatty acids, which our body is able to manufacture, and the essential fatty acids, which we have to supply to our body through our diet. These essential fatty acids are called unsaturated fats, and are liquid at room temperature.

Unsaturated fats are found in certain fish, nuts and vegetable oils, seeds, and soybeans especially, and, to some extent, in most foods. These essential fatty acids have been found to actually lower blood cholesterol.

Unsaturated Fats

Here are some foods that contain unsaturated fats:
- Bagels
- Barbecue sauce
- Bread

- Corn chips
- Fish (bluefish, cod, haddock, herring, mackerel, salmon, sardines, mussels, oysters, rainbow trout, scallops, and whitefish)
- Nuts (pine, walnuts, and Brazil)
- Popcorn (air-popped)
- Seeds
- Soybeans
- Squash
- Sweet potatoes
- Tofu

Be aware that unsaturated fats that are "hydrogenated" or "partially hydrogenated" become, in fact, saturated. Watch for these words when buying packaged foods.

Unfortunately, most fat ingested by the average American is of the nonessential, saturated variety. It is not necessary to consume any saturated fats in order to meet your "good" fat requirements—unsaturated fats provide everything you need. Saturated fats are contained in all meat and dairy products and are usually solid at room temperature. Remember that saturated fats raise total blood cholesterol.

Saturated Fats

Here are some foods high in saturated fat:
- Beef (fattier cuts)
- Butter
- Cheese
- Chocolate
- Coconut and all coconut products
- Cream
- Eggs (yolks)
- Fried foods (using saturated oils)
- Lard
- Lamb
- Pork
- Milk (whole, 2%, and 1%)
- Non-dairy creamers and non-dairy whipped cream
- Pork
- Sauces with a butter or cream base

- Turkey (dark meat)
- Veal

Over the past twenty years, American fat consumption has climbed from the recommended minimum of 20 percent to more than 40 percent in the average diet. Few of us realize how much hidden fat we consume. Knowing how much fat you eat is a key component in your quest for good health. Many other countries typically have lower levels of fat in their food than American cuisine, and eating ethnic dishes is a delicious way to lower the percentage of fat in your own diet as well. However, bear in mind that many restaurants serve portions large enough for two. If you are going to a restaurant you know dishes up hefty servings, ask for a half portion or take half home with you.

Common Fats and Oils

A Useful Table

Fat or Oil	Percent Saturated	Percent Unsaturated
Almond	8	92
Beef tallow	52	48
Butter (stick)	66	34
Canola	7	93
Chicken fat	30	70
Cocoa butter	62	38
Coconut	92	8
Corn	13	87
Cottonseed	27	73
Duck fat	34	66
Goose fat	27	73
Lard	41	59
Margarine (stick or whipped)	20	80
Olive	14	86
Palm	52	48
Palm kernel	87	13
Peanut	18	82
Safflower	9	91

Fat or Oil (cont.)	*Percent Saturated*	*Percent Unsaturated*
Salt pork fat	64	36
Sesame	15	85
Shortening (wheat germ)	27	73
Soybean	15	85
Soybean/cottonseed blend	19	81
Sunflower	11	89
Turkey fat	30	70
Walnut	14	86
Wheat germ	20	80

Lowest Saturated Fat: Canola, almond, and safflower oils
Highest Saturated Fat: Coconut and palm kernel oils, butter

SODIUM: Today most people know it's important to monitor their salt intake. The American Heart Association recommends a total salt intake of no more than 6 grams or 1½ teaspoons of salt per day. A high-salt diet will aggravate high blood pressure and cause bloating. Some recent studies suggest that sensitivity to salt increases with age as well. Many foods high in fat are also high in salt. If you are concerned about eating too much salt, stay away from foods that are pickled, smoked, in cocktail sauce, in broth, have soy sauce, or have MSG.

CARBOHYDRATES: There are two types of carbohydrates: simple and complex. Simple carbohydrates are easily digested by the body and provide energy quickly—these are also known as sugars, which dissolve easily and are in liquid form. These are not generally as healthy for you, however, as complex carbohydrates, or starches, which provide longer-lasting energy and more dietary fiber. Complex carbohydrates are an excellent source of energy, fiber, vitamins, and minerals. In addition, complex carbohydrates are released into the body more slowly than simple carbohydrates, which helps regulate blood sugar levels. Breads, pasta, grains, cereals, and some vegetables are examples of foods high in complex carbohydrates.

CHOLESTEROL: Cholesterol is a white, waxy, fatty substance found in all foods that come from animal sources, particularly organ meats. It is found in meat, dairy products, poultry, and fish. It is an essential element of our diet although we don't need a lot of it.

Cholesterol in the body is classified into two types: high-density lipoprotein (HDL) cholesterol and low-density lipoprotein (LDL) cholesterol. HDL cholesterol contains more proteins than fat. This type is often called the "good" cholesterol. LDL cholesterol contains more fat than protein. It is often called "bad" cholesterol. Diet plays an important role in regulating serum cholesterol levels. Eating a diet high in saturated fats and cholesterol appears to heighten LDL cholesterol levels and to lower HDL cholesterol levels. Similarly, a low-fat, high-fiber diet seems to have a lowering effect on LDL cholesterol and a heightening effect on HDL cholesterol. Other factors, such as activity level and genetics, also affect your total serum cholesterol level. While cholesterol helps build cell membranes, produce hormones, and manufacture acids that eliminate extra cholesterol from our bodies, eating too much cholesterol can cause clogged arteries, high blood pressure, strokes, and heart disease. Animal fats are the only fats that contain cholesterol and limiting your intake of these can reduce your total serum cholesterol. One word of caution: some tropical oils, such as coconut, palm, and palm kernel oil, can encourage the body to create more cholesterol even though these products are cholesterol-free.

FIBER: Fiber is plentiful in fruits, vegetables, beans, and grains. There are two types of dietary fiber: soluble and insoluble. Soluble fibers hold water and appear to reduce total blood cholesterol levels. Oats, beans, apples, and citrus fruits all provide soluble fiber.

Insoluble fiber is found in vegetables, whole grains, and bran. It helps move waste through your intestines, shortening the time harmful substances are in contact with your digestive tract. A diet high in insoluble fiber may reduce the risk of certain types of cancer, such as colorectal cancer.

Because they contain bulk and often few calories, high-fiber foods can help you feel full and maintain a healthy weight. A low-fat diet high in complex carbohydrates should provide all the fiber needed for good health.

The Cuisines

Ethnic restaurants are popular, convenient, and often inexpensive places to enjoy delicious, healthy meals. Their foreign, sometimes exotic settings, can foster the illusion of a trip abroad.

This book lists by section the most popular dishes and menus from a variety of major ethnic cuisines—African, Caribbean, Chinese, French, German and Austrian, Greek and Middle Eastern, Indian, Italian, Japanese, Mexican, Russian and Eastern European, Spanish, and Thai. Here you will find the ingredients of your favorite dishes and numerous menu options, including soups, appetizers, main dishes, side dishes, vegetables, and desserts. To help you choose menus that are both healthful and good-tasting, the book provides a detailed nutritional breakdown of your favorite dishes in terms of calories and serving size, as well as fat, sodium, carbohydrate, cholesterol, and fiber content. You can turn to this survey of ethnic cuisines for a broad array of dishes and menus along with the detailed nutritional information that will enable you to maintain a low-fat, low-cholesterol diet when you are dining at ethnic restaurants. Order wisely, control the size of your portions, select low-fat and low-calorie dishes—and enjoy the healthy pleasures of ethnic dining!

African Cuisine

African meals, in their variety of ingredients, can provide an abundance of vitamins and minerals, as well as an exciting change of pace for the typical American diner. This continent features a wide mix of legumes and fruits, and tracts of land ideal for raising livestock. Starches and vegetables served with a rich meat- or fish-based broth characterize African cooking. Fufus, or stiff puddings, are made by boiling starchy foods, such as yams, plantains, cassava or rice, and pounding them into a glutenous mass with an oversized mortar and pestle. They are a popular African staple and provide bulk with a minimum of fat. The same is true of rice, another popular side dish. The catch is, these are not served alone, but along with a flavorful soup, stew, or casserole, and this pervasive use of meaty sauces tends to increase fat counts. One way to cut down on fat and calories is to eat only a small amount of stew as an accent to your meal. (Strict vegetarians will want to exercise caution when ordering in African restaurants since vegetable dishes are often flavored with meat-based sauces.) Most fat-conscious diners will also want to avoid items which contain peanuts, peanut oil, or coconuts, and those that are deep-fried. If you are worried about the fat content of your meal, don't hesitate to ask what the dish contains and how it is prepared. It may be possible to change the method of cooking, or substitute ingredients, in order to lower the overall fat. On the whole, African dishes are some of the most varied and interesting available, especially to American palates, and if you avoid fatty meats and oils, they can be among the most healthful as well.

AFRICAN DISHES

FOOD NAME

Soups and Stews
Lowest Fat: *Fish Soup—18.4 g fat, 305.6 calories*
Highest Fat: *Sunday Stew—56.8 g fat, 659.3 calories*

BEAN SOUP *Gbegiri* with chicken stock, black-eyed beans, dry smoked fish, onion, tomato puree, and palm nut oil

BEEF AND VEGETABLE STEW *Taushe* with beef, tomatoes, pumpkin, onion, peanut oil, and chile powder

FISH SOUP *Alapa* with fish, lime juice, tomatoes, onion, chile powder, and cloves

OKRA SOUP with pork, okra, dry smoked fish, tomatoes, ground crayfish, and peanut oil

SUNDAY STEW with beef, tomatoes, onion, peanut oil, and chile powder

Side Dishes
Lowest Fat: *Rice Fufu—0.6 g fat, 264 calories*
Highest Fat: *Boiled Sweet Potatoes with Peanuts—44.2 g fat, 659.8 calories*

BLACK-EYED BEAN FRITTERS *Kosai-akara* with black-eyed beans, onion, and chile powder, deep-fried

BOILED SWEET POTATOES WITH PEANUTS *Dankali da geda* with sweet potatoes, peanuts, coconut, coconut milk, and spices

COCONUT AND SWEET CORN with coconut, corn, peanuts, coconut milk, chile peppers, butter, and spices

COUSCOUS semolina with chickpeas, lamb, turnips, carrots, zucchini, cabbage, and sweet peppers

DEEP-FRIED PLANTAINS *Ipekere*

FUFU, CORNMEAL *Ine-oka* stiff pudding of water and cornmeal

Serving Size	Calories	Fat (g)	Sodium (mg)	Carbohydrate (g)	Cholesterol (mg)	Fiber (g)
1 cup	577.8	34.8	**2903**	13.4	57	0.2
1½ cups	495.3	36.7	254.7	9	98	1.2
1½ cups	305.6	18.4	155.7	3.7	93.5	0.3
1½ cups	293.6	22.7	488.5	6.1	39.8	0.6
1½ cups	**659.3**	**56.8**	258.5	8.3	98	0.7
2 1-inch fritters	146.2	9.1	55.3	12.5	0	0.8
8 oz	**659.8**	**44.2**	21.4	50.6	0	3.4
3/4 cup	198	13.4	19.5	20.2	0	3.8
1 cup	335.5	16.5	308.9	31.2	45.2	3
5 oz (½ plantain)	179.8	10.4	3	23.6	0	0.4
1 cup	427.1	4	1.1	88	0	1.2

AFRICAN DISHES

FOOD NAME

FUFU, RICE *Rice Tuwo* stiff pudding of water and rice

FUFU, YAM FLOUR stiff pudding of water and yam flour

Meat and Poultry
Lowest Fat: *Chopone–Choptwo—17.8 g fat, 308.4 calories*
Highest Fat: *Pork Pineapple—55.4 g fat, 720 calories*

CHICKEN DRUMSTICKS chicken drumsticks deep-fried with peanuts and chili powder

CURRIED MEAT TRIANGLES with mutton, onion, and short-crust pastry, fried in oil

CHOPONE–CHOPTWO pastry with shredded beef, onion, and sweet pepper

PEPPER CHICKEN with chicken breasts, onion, tomatoes, and chili powder

PORK PINEAPPLE with fried pork, onion and cayenne pepper

STUFFED VEGETABLES with onions, tomatoes, green peppers, and rice, bread crumbs, corned beef, and pork

Desserts
Lowest Fat: *Niger Pineapple—5.5 g fat, 237.5 calories*
Highest Fat: *Banana Fritters—28.2 g fat, 451.2 calories*

BANANA FRITTERS deep-fried, with sugar, flour and egg white

MANGO SLICE with mango, custard, and pastry

NIGER PINEAPPLE with condensed milk, gelatin, and pineapple juice

PAWPAW FOOL with sugar, vanilla custard, and whipped cream

Serving Size	Calories	Fat (g)	Sodium (mg)	Carbohydrate (g)	Cholesterol (mg)	Fiber (g)
1 cup	264	0.6	4	57.2	0	0.2
1 cup	462.9	0.7	42.6	87.8	0	1.5
1 drumstick	231.9	18.3	167.9	1.2	59	0.2
2 2-oz triangles	**525.6**	46.8	256.9	7.3	133.9	0.1
2 2-oz triangles	308.4	17.8	149.3	7.8	135.3	0.2
1 4-oz breast	442.4	33.6	115.2	3.4	97.2	0.3
8 oz	**720**	**55.4**	145.5	15.5	169	0.8
8 oz	316.7	14.6	**998.8**	10.1	**734**	0.9
1 cup	**451.2**	**28.2**	72.7	41.8	0	0.7
1 cup	**497.8**	23.2	343.2	57.4	320.8	1.2
1 cup	237.5	5.5	78.3	43.5	23.8	0.3
1 cup	278.4	14.7	159.6	32.4	167.2	0.6

AFRICAN DISHES

FOOD NAME

Beverages
Lowest Fat: Pineapple Drink—0.3 g fat, 74.4 calories
Highest Fat: Orange Shake—8.3 g fat, 163.3 calories

FRUIT PUNCH   with oranges, pineapple, pawpaw, guavas, and lemonade

ORANGE SHAKE   with orange juice, milk, and vanilla ice cream

PINEAPPLE DRINK   *Chinanadzi*   with pineapple, ginger, cloves, and sugar

Serving Size	Calories	Fat (g)	Sodium (mg)	Carbohydrate (g)	Cholesterol (mg)	Fiber (g)
1 cup	124.7	0.3	1.9	30.9	1	0.7
1 cup	163.3	8.3	62.4	18	31.2	0.1
1 cup	74.4	0.3	1	17.9	1.5	0.2

Caribbean Cuisine

The wonderful thing about Caribbean cuisine is that every one of the islands and island groups has unique dishes due to the variety of ethnic food influences in this region. Over the centuries, an eclectic assortment of culinary traditions have prevailed, including: Dutch, East Indian, French, Native American, English, and especially African and Spanish foods. The word "créole" is often used to describe Caribbean cooking because the islands feature such a healthy mix of peoples from around the globe. The result is a delicious medley of different tastes. Fish dishes are in abundance on many Caribbean menus and are a good low-fat choice for diners as long as the dish is steamed or poached rather than fried. Some popular exotic ingredients used in Caribbean cuisine include breadfruit, okra, papaya, yucca, and star fruit (carambola). As in Thai food, coconut is used in many dishes—the fat-conscious diner should avoid these dishes since coconut is very high in fat. Coconut oil or lard, both of which are loaded with saturated fat, are traditionally used to prepare many Caribbean dishes, so be sure to ask your server what type of oil is used in fried or sautéed dishes. Better yet, avoid fried foods and choose a more healthful curry or poached fish. Then if you want to avoid additional calories, top off your delicious meal with a tasty fruit drink (without the alcohol) instead of those mango fritters!

CARIBBEAN DISHES

FOOD NAME

Appetizers
Lowest Fat: Plantain Chips—14.2 g fat, 301 calories
Highest Fat: Yam Fritters—42.2 g fat, 508.8 calories

BANANA FRITTERS *Banana Accras* with bananas, flour, milk, and egg, fried in vegetable oil

PLANTAIN CHIPS *Plátanos Fritos* plantains fried in vegetable oil

SHRIMP FRITTERS *Shrimp Accras* shrimp with flour, curry powder, scallions, and green peppers, fried in vegetable oil

YAM FRITTERS *Yam Accras* with yams, eggs, parsley, scallions, and chile peppers, fried in vegetable oil

Soups and Side Dishes
Lowest Fat: Callaloo Soup—8.3 g fat, 236.7 calories
Highest Fat: Calabaza—34.5 g fat, 400.2 calories

BLACK BEANS AND RICE *Moros y Cristianos* with black beans, rice, onion, red bell peppers, tomato, garlic, and chile peppers

CALLALOO SOUP with Swiss chard, corned beef, crab, okra, coconut milk, garlic, and onion

CALABAZA *Colombo de Giraumon* with West Indian pumpkin, salt pork, bell peppers, and curry powder

SHRIMP BISQUE with shrimp, half-and-half, sweet butter, chile peppers, salt, and pepper

PEPPERPOT SOUP with beef, pork, spinach, scallions, white yam, okra, and cilantro

RICE WITH VEGETABLE SAUCE with rice, onions, bell peppers, tomatoes, cabbage, and cilantro

Serving Size	Calories	Fat (g)	Sodium (mg)	Carbohydrate (g)	Cholesterol (mg)	Fiber (g)
1 cup	295.9	16.4	80.7	29.3	71	0.5
1 cup	301	14.2	539	47.2	0	0.7
1 cup	384	21.2	**690**	20.4	81.8	0.4
1 cup	**508.8**	**42.2**	353.8	28	156.6	1.1
1½ cups	334	11.1	279.4	50.5	0	0.7
1 cup	236.7	8.3	**983.1**	14.9	35.6	0.5
1 cup	**400.2**	**34.5**	744.9	22.7	32	1.9
1 cup	387.8	32.6	337.3	10.6	178.5	0.1
1 cup	213.4	10	309.7	10.4	49.2	0.6
1½ cups	327	8.4	265.7	57.4	20.7	0.7

CARIBBEAN DISHES

FOOD NAME

Meat and Poultry
Lowest Fat: Stuffed Cho-Cho—7.5 g fat, 254.4 calories
Highest Fat: Stuffed Plantains—85.4 g fat, 1043.1 calories

CHICKEN COLOMBO   with chicken, ginger, turmeric, curry powder, cinnamon, cardamom, allspice, chile peppers, garlic, and onions

CHICKEN STEW   *Sancocho*   with chicken, lime juice, celery, scallions, bell peppers, onions, tomatoes, nutmeg, cumin, carrots, plantains, calabaza, yam, cabbage, and corn

LAMB WITH BEANS AND RICE   lamb with beans, rice, garlic and Sofrito powder

PAPAYA BEEF STEAK   beef with papaya, onions, tomato, lentils, and chile peppers

STUFFED CHO-CHO   Chayote squash with beef round, red bell peppers, tomato paste, and parsley

STUFFED PLANTAINS   *Piononos*   plantains with ground chuck, ham, scallions, tomatoes, and capers, fried in vegetable oil

Seafood
Lowest Fat: Crayfish—1.5 g fat, 149.4 calories
Highest Fat: Red Snapper Curaçao-Style—18.7 g fat, 447.3 calories

WHITE FISH IN BROTH   *Blaff*   with white fish, lime, garlic, chile peppers, white wine, scallions, and cilantro

SKEWERED CONCH   *Brochette de Lambi*   Conch with smoked bacon, chayote, onion, garlic, celery leaves, and thyme

SPICY SPINY LOBSTER   lobster with onions, limes, tomatoes, bay leaves, celery and chile peppers

CRAYFISH   *Ouassous au nage*   Crayfish with onions, bell peppers, cilantro, lime juice, and vinegar

RED SNAPPER CURAÇAO-STYLE   red snapper with bell peppers, tomatoes, lime juice, garlic, chile peppers, flour, and butter

Serving Size	Calories	Fat (g)	Sodium (mg)	Carbohydrate (g)	Cholesterol (mg)	Fiber (g)
1½ cups	725.5	46	674.5	6.3	291.5	0.4
1½ cups	455.1	18.3	544.1	26.1	147.5	1.2
1½ cups	555	31.1	313.9	50.7	45	0.7
8 oz	536	33.5	215.6	21.6	110.3	1.5
8 oz (½ stuffed squash)	254.4	7.5	144.4	33	34.6	2.8
2 4-oz patties	**1043.1**	**85.4**	**1048.4**	42.3	317.7	1.2
8 oz	321.6	13.4	**924**	5.7	135.2	0.2
1½ cups	313.6	10	**1054.9**	20.2	88.1	0.9
1 1¼-pound lobster	397.4	16.3	**920**	11.4	243	0.8
1½ cups	149.4	1.5	633.3	10.2	121.5	0.4
8 oz	447.3	18.7	390.5	15.7	116.3	1

CARIBBEAN DISHES

FOOD NAME

SHRIMP AND RICE   shrimp with rice, bell peppers, carrots, scallions, celery, butter, parsley, nutmeg, and chili powder

Beverages
Lowest Fat: Ginger Beer—0 g fat, 47.8 calories
Highest Fat: Planter's Punch—0.2 g fat, 303.9 calories

DAIQUIRI, BANANA   with fresh fruit, banana liqueur, and cream

DAIQUIRI, STRAWBERRY   with rum, fresh strawberries, honey, and cream

GINGER BEER   with ginger root, lime, cream of tartar, and sugar

PLANTER'S PUNCH   with rum, lime juice, orange juice, and sugar

SHRUB   with light rum, orange zest, vanilla bean, cinnamon, and cane sugar syrup

Desserts
Lowest Fat: Guava Paste Turnovers—11.3 g fat, 295.7 calories
Highest Fat: Coconut Ice Cream—23.6 g fat, 278.5 calories

COCONUT ICE CREAM   with almond extract and dark rum

GUAVA PASTE TURNOVERS   *Empanadas* with flour, sugar, butter, egg yolk, vanilla extract, nutmeg, and cinnamon

KEY LIME PIE   with eggs, sweetened condensed milk, lime juice, and sugar

MANGO FRITTERS   with mango, flour, milk, sugar, lemon juice, and vanilla extract, fried in vegetable oil

Serving Size	Calories	Fat (g)	Sodium (mg)	Carbohydrate (g)	Cholesterol (mg)	Fiber (g)
1½ cups	399.5	9.6	285.6	57.8	129	0.8
8 oz	289.1	4.8	6.4	23.2	16.6	0.1
9½ oz	359.7	5.2	8.1	40.2	16.6	0.8
8 oz	47.8	0	1.0	12.4	0	0
6 oz	**303.9**	0.2	6.3	24.2	0	0
2 oz	151.5	0	0	3	0	0
½ cup	**278.5**	**23.6**	71	14	73.4	1
2 3-inch half-moon turnovers	295.7	11.3	141.5	40	71.2	2.6
1 4-inch slice	**499**	20.8	299.5	59.4	272	0.1
2 2-oz fritters	254.5	14.4	**70.4**	22.3	94.1	0.5

Chinese Cuisine

Chinese food can be either very nutritious or very naughty, depending on what dishes you select. Two red flags to watch for when eating Chinese are fried foods and high-sodium soups and sauces. Anything called "sweet-and-sour" or "crispy" is usually deep-fried. Monosodium glutamate, or MSG, is a sodium-based flavor enhancer used commonly (but not exclusively) in Asian restaurants. It is usually present unless specified otherwise, so request an MSG-free meal to avoid ingesting excessive amounts of sodium. Chinese soups tend to be full of salt as well. Many foods that are low in fat, such as vegetables, are often served with high-fat garnishes. These foods are denoted on the menu with such phrases as "with egg" and "with almonds." Most restaurants will be happy to accommodate you if you ask for plain vegetables, without the extras. Servings are often large enough to accommodate two, so don't feel you have to eat everything on your plate. Rice contains bulky complex carbohydrates which take time for your system to break down, so eating a good amount of rice during the meal will help you feel satisfied longer. It is also a much healthier, lower-fat way to fill up than ingesting a heap of sweet-and-sour chicken or barbecued pork. If possible, choose brown rice over white. While enriched white rice offers as much or even more than brown rice in the way of vitamins and minerals, a cup of cooked brown rice contains four times more dietary fiber (1.6 grams, as opposed to .4 grams) than polished, or white, rice. Both types are good sources of protein.

CHINESE DISHES

FOOD NAME

Appetizers
Lowest Fat: *Steamed Vegetable Dumplings—0.6 g fat, 65.5 calories*
Highest Fat: *Egg Roll—29 g fat, 407.6 calories*

BARBECUED SPARERIBS *Shao P'ai Ku* Spare ribs with hoisin sauce, soy sauce, sesame oil, five-spice powder, and brown sugar

COLD SESAME NOODLES noodles with sesame oil, soy sauce, garlic, sesame paste, cider vinegar, and sugar

EGG ROLL minced pork with vegetables, deep-fried in rice paper wrapping

FRIED WONTONS *Cha Yün T'un* with Chinese cabbage, ground pork, scallions, ginger, soy sauce, sherry, chicken broth, and egg

PLUM-FLAVORED PORK TENDERLOIN pork marinated and roasted with plums, hoisin sauce, soy sauce, sesame oil, ginger, orange and lemon juice

POTSTICKER DUMPLINGS with flour dough, Chinese cabbage, ground pork, scallions, ginger, sherry, soy sauce, and sesame oil, pan-fried and served with soy dipping sauce

SHRIMP AND PORK DUMPLINGS Shrimp with cilantro, sesame oil, and cornstarch in wonton skins, steamed and served with soy-vinegar dip

SHRIMP BALLS *Hsia Ch'iu* made with egg, bread, shrimp, water chestnuts, soy sauce, sesame oil, and cornstarch

SHRIMP TOAST *Mien Pao Hsia* made with shrimp, French bread, scallions, egg, and sesame seeds, deep-fried in vegetable oil

SOY-BRAISED CHICKEN WINGS with chicken, scallions, ginger, sherry, and mushroom soy sauce

SPRING ROLLS egg and flour wrappers filled with pork, scallions, bamboo shoots, Chinese cabbage, bean sprouts, and carrots, deep-fried and served with soy-vinegar dip

Serving Size	Calories	Fat (g)	Sodium (mg)	Carbohydrate (g)	Cholesterol (mg)	Fiber (g)
3 1-oz ribs	383.4	13.2	**2145.4**	39.0	36.3	0
¾ cup	243.1	12.2	**1048.2**	28.8	0	0.4
1 egg roll	**407.6**	**29**	469.5	21.2	96.9	0.6
4 wontons	294.4	20.9	227.2	20.7	36.5	0.2
8 oz	395.6	26.2	676	17.2	64.8	0.3
3 dumplings	173	10.2	**637**	14.8	10.3	0.2
3 dumplings	269	10.8	**1008**	29.8	59	0.1
2 balls	188.6	9.6	366.5	10.8	120.9	0.1
3 2-inch toasts	388.4	22.5	533.9	25.7	161.2	0.1
3 wings (4 ounces total)	174.1	11.5	67.2	4.1	47.5	.03
1 spring roll	221.6	18.1	**974.7**	11.2	8.1	0.3

CHINESE DISHES

FOOD NAME

STEAMED VEGETABLE DUMPLINGS with flour, mushrooms, egg, scallions, bamboo shoots, carrot, garlic, sherry, soy sauce, salt, MSG and sugar.

STEAMED SHRIMP DUMPLINGS *Har Kow* made with water chestnuts, scallions, soy sauce, and sesame oil in wheat dough, steamed and served with soy-vinegar dip

Soups
Lowest Fat: Bean Curd Soup—3.9 g fat, 80.2 calories
Highest Fat: Sizzling Rice Soup—11 g fat, 258 calories

BEAN CURD SOUP with Chinese mushrooms, chicken stock, carrots, scallions, soy sauce, and cilantro

CHINESE CABBAGE SOUP with onion, ginger, Chinese cabbage, soy sauce, and sesame oil

EGG DROP SOUP *Chi Tan T'ang* with chicken stock, soy sauce, ginger, eggs, scallions, and sesame oil

HOT-AND-SOUR SOUP with pork, Chinese mushrooms, chicken stock, bamboo shoots, water chestnuts, bean curd, spices and egg

NOODLE SOUP WITH FISH AND SPINACH WONTONS with wheat flour noodles, chicken stock, flounder filets, spinach, scallions, and sesame oil

NOODLE SOUP WITH PORK WONTONS AND CHINESE ROAST PORK with pork, wheat flour noodles, chicken broth, snow peas, and scallions

SHARK FIN SOUP with scallions, ginger, chicken stock, chicken breast, egg whites, sherry, and cornstarch

SIZZLING RICE SOUP with Chinese mushrooms, bamboo shoots, eggs, chicken broth, and deep-fried white rice

VELVET CORN SOUP with corn, scallions, ginger, sherry, chicken stock, and egg whites

Serving Size	Calories	Fat (g)	Sodium (mg)	Carbohydrate (g)	Cholesterol (mg)	Fiber (g)
5 dumplings	65.5	0.6	124.5	12.6	18.3	.30
3 dumplings	344	9	736	38.7	115.6	0.4
1 cup	80.2	3.9	773.1	3.4	0.5	0.3
1 cup	66.3	5.7	579	3.7	0	0.3
1 cup	109.6	7.1	588.9	2.7	219.8	.02
1 cup	131.5	8.1	749.2	4.8	59.7	0.3
1 cup	353.6	5.6	674.2	49.2	41.7	0.2
1 cup	297.3	6.2	717.3	42.2	41.7	0.2
1 cup	129.6	4.8	**1152.8**	4.1	16.5	0.2
1 cup	**258**	**11**	851	30.5	69.3	0.1
1 cup	159	6.6	609.7	17.8	110.2	0.5

CHINESE DISHES

FOOD NAME

WINTER MELON SOUP   with winter melon, Chinese mushrooms, chicken breast, pork, ham, water chestnuts, chicken stock, and eggs

WONTON SOUP   made with water chestnuts, pork, ginger, sesame oil, egg, wonton skins, soy sauce, and chicken stock

Poultry
Lowest Fat: Chicken, Broccoli, and Water Chestnuts in Oyster Sauce—9 g fat, 195.3 calories
Highest Fat: Peking Duck—112 g fat, 2061.8 calories

BEGGAR'S CHICKEN   with ground pork, ginger, pickled mustard greens, soy sauce, sherry, sesame oil, and lotus leaves, cooked in a flour crust

CHICKEN WITH BROCCOLI   with chicken breasts, chicken broth, peanut oil, garlic, cornstarch, sugar, salt and MSG

CHICKEN, BROCCOLI, AND WATER CHESTNUTS IN OYSTER SAUCE   with sherry, garlic, ginger, soy sauce, and chicken broth

CHICKEN WITH CASHEWS   chicken with cornstarch, soy sauce, white wine, chicken broth, scallions, and sesame oil

DUCK BRAISED WITH BAMBOO SHOOTS, CHESTNUTS, AND MUSHROOMS   duck with bamboo shoots, mushrooms, chestnuts, cinnamon, cloves, fennel, anise, tangerine peel, and sherry

DRUNKEN CHICKEN   chicken with ginger, five-spice powder, scallions, and sherry

EMPRESS CHICKEN   chicken with Chinese mushrooms, ginger, scallions, sherry, soy sauce, brown sugar, and bamboo shoots

HOISIN CHICKEN   diced chicken with cornstarch, sherry, ginger, garlic, scallions, hoisin sauce, soy sauce, chicken broth, and sesame oil

Serving Size	Calories	Fat (g)	Sodium (mg)	Carbohydrate (g)	Cholesterol (mg)	Fiber (g)
1 cup	179.1	7.3	648.6	7.9	117.5	0.4
1¼ cups	186.7	6.2	709	22.7	50.4	0.1
8 oz	691	51.5	499.7	1.5	213.4	.02
1 cup	376.4	24.0	387.7	7.1	92.1	.50
½ cup	195.3	9	**961.4**	8.3	48.7	0.3
⅔ cup	322	21.8	499.6	7.6	54.9	0.3
1¾ cups	**1068**	**91**	**1520**	23.1	174.4	0.9
8 oz	871	34	**1736**	12.4	198.6	0.1
1 cup	577	38	**1546**	6.4	180.3	0.3
1 cup	705.6	31.8	**2340.4**	30.6	146.2	0.2

CHINESE DISHES

FOOD NAME

KUNG PAO CHICKEN chicken with egg, cornstarch, rice, vinegar, sherry, bell peppers, scallions, ginger, hot peppers, and sesame oil

LEMON CHICKEN chicken with soy sauce, ginger, lemon zest and juice, chicken broth, and sesame oil

PEKING DUCK *Peiching K'ao Ya* duck with honey, scallions, hoisin sauce, and soy sauce, and served with Mu Shu Pancakes (see also Mu Shu Pancakes, page 44)

PINEAPPLE DUCK IN GINGER FRUIT SAUCE with duck breast, soy sauce, cornstarch, candied and fresh ginger, bell peppers, sherry, and sesame oil

SHREDDED CHICKEN WITH TREE EARS AND MUSHROOMS shredded chicken with tree ears, mushrooms, cornstarch, soy sauce, sherry, ginger, and scallions

SHREDDED COLD CHICKEN WITH HOT PEANUT DRESSING shredded chicken with peanut butter, cayenne pepper, ginger, garlic, sesame oil, and cider vinegar

SPICY CHICKEN WITH PEANUTS AND BAMBOO SHOOTS chicken with egg white, peanuts, bamboo shoots, scallions, ginger, garlic, chicken broth, and sesame oil

SWEET-AND-SOUR CHICKEN chicken, deep-fried in batter with pineapple and sweet-and-sour sauce

TEA-SMOKED CHICKEN chicken with soy sauce, ginger, scallions, cinnamon, anise, rice, and sesame oil

Beef Dishes
Lowest Fat: *Beef with Oyster Sauce—21.1 g fat, 337.9 calories*
Highest Fat: *Orange Beef—65.7 g fat, 819.2 calories*

ANTS CLIMBING A TREE with bean threads, scallions, ground beef, chicken stock, sherry, soy sauce, chili paste, and sesame oil

Serving Size	Calories	Fat (g)	Sodium (mg)	Carbohydrate (g)	Cholesterol (mg)	Fiber (g)
1 cup	720.2	54.2	**1437.9**	16	165.8	0.7
8 oz	482	36	**1522**	2	149.5	0
12 oz	**2061.8**	**112**	**2297.4**	**184.4**	**203.9**	**1.9**
1¼ cups	906.4	80.7	626.8	18	133.1	0.6
½ cup	186.4	9.2	400.2	3.6	54.8	0.2
1 cup	910	65	760	5.3	**234**	0.5
1 cup	474	34	449	9.7	78.1	0.7
1¼ cups	620	39.1	408.4	43.2	65.8	0.6
12 ounces	817	51	**3010**	15.6	**263.7**	0.1
1 cup	680	57.3	821.3	7.1	128.3	.06

CHINESE DISHES

FOOD NAME

BEEF WITH OYSTER SAUCE beef with soy sauce, cornstarch, sherry, ginger, and scallions

BROCCOLI WITH BEEF with beef, broccoli, soy sauce, cornstarch, ginger, sugar, and brandy

GINGER BEEF with flank steak, soy sauce, sherry, cornstarch, fresh ginger, scallions, and sesame oil

HOT AND SPICY SHREDDED BEEF shredded beef with ginger, carrots, scallions, soy sauce, hoisin sauce, yellow bean sauce, chili paste, sherry, and sesame oil

HUNAN BEEF ON A BED OF SPINACH beef with spinach, ginger, scallions, anise, cinnamon, hot peppers, sherry, and soy sauce

ORANGE BEEF beef with soy sauce, ginger, orange zest and juice, sherry, hoisin sauce, and sesame oil, fried in vegetable oil

OXTAIL STEW Oxtails with soy sauce, beef broth, ginger, tomato paste, oyster sauce, sherry, and cilantro

Pork Dishes
Lowest Fat: *Braised Bean Threads, Pork, and Vegetables—14 g fat, 223 calories*
Highest Fat: *Sweet and Sour Pork—62.5 g fat, 719.5 calories*

BRAISED BEAN THREADS, PORK, AND VEGETABLES pork with tree ears (fungi), bean threads, Chinese mushrooms, sherry, chicken stock, turnips, bok choy, and leeks

MU SHU PORK pork with Chinese mushrooms, water chestnuts, cornstarch, soy sauce, white wine, eggs, scallions, and ginger, wrapped in pancakes and served with hoisin sauce

RED ROAST PORK *Char Sui* pork with soy sauce, hoisin sauce, ketchup, sherry, garlic, five-spice powder, and brown sugar

SHREDDED PORK, BAMBOO SHOOTS, AND GREEN PEPPER IN BLACK BEAN SAUCE with cornstarch, white wine, soy sauce, cider vinegar, ginger and sherry

Serving Size	Calories	Fat (g)	Sodium (mg)	Carbohydrate (g)	Cholesterol (mg)	Fiber (g)
1 cup	450.5	28.1	**1504.5**	15.5	79.3	.06
1 cup	171.9	13.9	422.1	4.2	14.9	0.4
1 cup	490.5	35.9	796.1	8.7	79.3	0.3
1 cup	514.7	34.7	**2300**	15.2	105.1	1.2
12 oz	702	52	718	8	155.5	0.9
1 cup	**819.2**	**65.7**	938.9	20.3	105.3	0.1
1½ cups	720.2	52.3	**1447.8**	10.7	135.4	0.4
1¼ cups	223	14	905	14	27.6	1.7
two 6-inch filled pancake rolls	582.4	39.2	906.4	35.4	255.7	0.6
8 oz	697	52	**2369**	16.4	164.5	.05
1 cup	617.7	42.9	969.6	12.9	135.1	0.5

CHINESE DISHES

FOOD NAME

SPICY BEAN CURD WITH GROUND PORK   bean curd with white wine, scallions, soy sauce, chili paste, and sugar

SWEET-AND-SOUR PORK   *T'ang Ts'u Chu Jo*   pork deep-fried with egg, cornstarch, ginger, bell peppers, soy sauce, vinegar, and ketchup

SZECHUAN PORK   *Ch'uan Jo*   pork with fermented black beans, garlic, scallions, sherry, soy sauce, chili paste, hoisin sauce, and tomato paste

Fish and Shellfish Dishes
Lowest Fat: *Drunken Shrimp—4 g fat, 377 calories*
Highest Fat: *Kung Pao Shrimp—31 g fat, 466 calories*

CLAMS WITH BLACK BEAN SAUCE   clams with garlic, black beans, and soy sauce

CRABMEAT OMELET   *Hsich Jo Chi Ton*   with crabmeat, egg, Chinese mushrooms, water chestnuts, bamboo shoots, ginger, scallions, and bean sprouts

DRUNKEN SHRIMP   shrimp with sherry, brandy, ginger, scallions, vinegar, soy sauce, sugar, and ginger oil

FIREPOT HONG KONG STYLE   *Huo Kuo*   with bean threads, chicken breast, filet mignon, calf's liver, flounder, lobster, shrimp, oysters, clams, mussels, Chinese cabbage, meat stock, and sherry

KUNG PAO SHRIMP   with shrimp, egg, scallions, ginger, garlic, hot red peppers, peanuts, sherry, and sesame oil

LOBSTER WITH SCALLIONS AND GINGER   with lobster, soy sauce, sherry, chicken broth, and sesame oil

SHRIMP WITH GARLIC SAUCE   with large shrimp, garlic, soy sauce, sesame oil, scallions, shao hsing sauce, salt, sugar and MSG

SHRIMP OMELET WITH CHINESE BROWN SAUCE   with shrimp, ginger, scallions, celery, bell peppers, and bean sprouts

Serving Size	Calories	Fat (g)	Sodium (mg)	Carbohydrate (g)	Cholesterol (mg)	Fiber (g)
¾ cup	416	32	**1369.3**	6.3	54.8	1.7
1 cup	719.5	**62.5**	831.7	12.6	155.3	0.1
1 cup	780	62	671	10.8	164.5	0.4
9 clams	198.7	7	185.4	5.7	60	.03
10 oz	362.0	26.4	**1161.2**	5.6	**571.3**	1.6
8 oz	377	4	**1120**	7.6	346.7	.05
12 oz	472	18	821	11.9	320.7	0.9
¾ cup	466	**31**	693	15.2	241.8	0.9
½ medium lobster	414.4	31.1	**1279.8**	6.8	121.6	0.4
7 oz	510.7	38.8	**2328.5**	7.9	216.7	.15
8 oz	277.6	16.3	735	7	389.7	0.7

CHINESE DISHES

FOOD NAME

SPICY VELVET SHRIMP WITH CUCUMBERS AND PEAS   with shrimp, egg white, cornstarch, soy sauce, ginger, scallions, hot red peppers, peas, cucumbers, white wine, and chicken broth

STEAMED BLACK SEA BASS   *Chen Lu-Yü*   sea bass with scallions, ginger, soy sauce, sherry, and sesame oil

VELVET SHRIMP WITH CASHEWS   shrimp with cashews, egg white, ginger, scallion, garlic, sherry, soy sauce, and chicken broth

Vegetable Dishes
Lowest Fat: *Braised Mixed Vegetables—3.7 g fat, 95.9 calories*
Highest Fat: *Vegetable Mu Shu—36 g fat, 579 calories*

BRAISED MIXED VEGETABLES   with bean threads, tree ears (fungi), Chinese mushrooms, ginger, bamboo shoots, corn, mushrooms, soy sauce, chicken broth, and sesame oil

BROCCOLI WITH OYSTER SAUCE   with broccoli, ginger, sugar, brandy, and sesame oil

BUDDHA'S DELIGHT   *Lo Hon Chai*   with bean curd, tree ears (fungi), bean threads, Chinese cabbage, carrot, celery, bamboo shoots, peanuts, soy sauce, and sesame oil

EGGPLANT IN SPICY GARLIC MEAT SAUCE   with eggplant, ground pork, soy sauce, ginger, scallions, chicken broth, chili paste, and sesame oil

SLOW-COOKED CHINESE CABBAGE   with cabbage, chicken stock, sesame oil, and sugar

SNOW PEAS WITH WATER CHESTNUTS   with snow peas, water chestnuts, and sesame seeds

SPICY GREEN BEANS   with green beans, fermented black beans, chili paste, garlic, ginger, green beans, and chicken broth

Serving Size	Calories	Fat (g)	Sodium (mg)	Carbohydrate (g)	Cholesterol (mg)	Fiber (g)
¾ cup	480	30.7	412	14.1	231.2	1
8 oz	250	8	416	1.3	181.3	0.1
¾ cup	445.6	24.4	659.1	14.9	322.4	0.4
⅔ cup	95.9	3.7	540	14.5	.1	0.8
½ cup	70.4	3.9	540.7	8.1	0	0.4
1 cup	362	35	807	8.5	0	1
½ cup	285	20	508	19.5	20.6	0.7
¾ cup	87	8	672	1.9	0.5	0.3
¾ cup	128	5	345	17.5	0	1.8
¾ cup	99	7	602	6.9	0.1	0.7

CHINESE DISHES

FOOD NAME

STIR-FRIED BEAN CURD WITH OYSTER SAUCE AND VEGETABLES bean curd with Chinese mushrooms, sherry, soy sauce, ginger, bok choy, bamboo shoots, baby corn, and sesame oil

SWEET-AND-SOUR CABBAGE cabbage with onion, soy sauce, white wine, cider vinegar, sugar, and hot red pepper

VEGETABLE MU SHU with Chinese mushrooms, eggs, water chestnuts, bean curd, bamboo shoots, soy sauce, sherry, bean sprouts, scallions, ginger, and hoisin sauce, served with Mu Shu Pancakes (see page 44)

Sauces & Staples
Lowest Fat: Soy Sauce—0 g fat, 11 calories
Highest Fat: Spicy Dipping Sauce—14 g fat, 242 calories

DUCK SAUCE with sweet bean paste, hoisin sauce, sugar, and sesame oil

MU SHU PANCAKES with flour, water, and sesame oil

MUSTARD SAUCE with sugar and vinegar

PEANUT HOISIN DIP with peanut butter, hoisin sauce, soy sauce, sesame oil, lemon juice, and Tabasco sauce

RICE, BROWN

RICE, WHITE

SOY SAUCE

SOY-VINEGAR DIP with ginger and sugar

SPICY DIPPING SAUCE with soy sauce, chile oil, sesame oil, scallions, and garlic

SWEET-AND-SOUR SAUCE with Chinese plum sauce and rice vinegar

Serving Size	Calories	Fat (g)	Sodium (mg)	Carbohydrate (g)	Cholesterol (mg)	Fiber (g)
1¼ cups	248	17	497	17.8	3.8	1.6
½ cup	164	10	748	17.6	0	1
2 filled pancake rolls	**579**	**36**	796	44.5	274	1.5
2 tablespoons	179.8	3.9	403	22.9	0	0.2
2 pancakes	84	3	0	12.6	0	0.5
2 tablespoons	78	6	5	4	0	0
2 tablespoons	70.4	5	157.0	4.6	0	0.2
1 cup cooked	352	.8	8	76	0	0.8
1 cup cooked	354	0.8	5	78.5	0	0.2
2 tablespoons	22	0	**2058**	3	0	0
2 tablespoons	18.1	0	**1372.3**	3.1	0	.03
2 tablespoons	53.4	3.4	**2058.3**	3.3	0	.03
2 tablespoons	291	3	0	70.1	0	3.2

CHINESE DISHES

FOOD NAME

Rice and Noodles

Lowest Fat: Bean Curd, Mushrooms, and Bok Choy with Noodles—6.5 g fat, 277.5 calories

Highest Fat: Chicken Chow Mein—53.4 g fat, 739.6 calories

BEAN CURD, MUSHROOMS, AND BOK CHOY WITH NOODLES

BRAISED NOODLES WITH CHICKEN with noodles, chicken, Chinese mushrooms, scallions, ginger, bok choy, sherry, soy sauce, chicken stock, and sesame oil

CHICKEN RICE CASSEROLE with chicken, rice, ginger, garlic, scallions, soy sauce, sherry, chicken broth, sausage, and cilantro

CHOW MEIN, BEEF wheat-flour noodles with steak, bean sprouts, bamboo shoots, and cabbage

CHOW MEIN, BEEF AND GREEN PEPPER wheat-flour noodles with soy sauce, sherry, scallions, ginger, garlic, chicken broth, oyster sauce, and ketchup

CHOW MEIN, CHICKEN egg noodles with chicken, shrimp, spinach, mushrooms, and water chestnuts

CHOW MEIN, PORK wheat-flour noodles with bean sprouts, bamboo shoots, and cabbage

EGG FOO YONG omelet with scallions, bean sprouts, ham, mushrooms, celery, and ginger, sprinkled with soy sauce

FRIED RICE, ASSORTED MEAT with ham, crabmeat, eggs, chicken, bamboo shoots, mushrooms, peas, and onions

FRIED RICE, PEAS AND HAM with rice, peas, ham, ginger and scallions

FRIED RICE, PORK with rice, pork, oil, scallions, salt, egg, soy sauce, and coriander

Serving Size	Calories	Fat (g)	Sodium (mg)	Carbohydrate (g)	Cholesterol (mg)	Fiber (g)
1½ cups	277.5	6.5	**1061**	44	0.8	0.9
1½ cups	677	22	**1212**	82.1	39.5	0.3
1½ cups	680	30.5	**1289.9**	36.6	188.5	0.2
1¼ cups	648	47.2	747.3	36.6	39.7	1.6
1¼ cups	662	22	495	82.2	31.8	0.4
1¼ cups	**739.6**	**53.4**	315.6	37.1	84.6	0.2
1¼ cups	710.9	52.3	745.4	36.6	67.6	1.6
10 oz	383.6	26.4	**1858.4**	13.9	**670.6**	1.9
1½ cups	507	20.8	**1125.4**	55.5	154.1	1.1
1½ cups	462.2	21.4	963.5	50.3	221.7	1.1
1½ cups	447.1	22.4	**1255.6**	45.3	224.5	0.4

CHINESE DISHES

FOOD NAME

FRIED RICE, SHRIMP with rice, shrimp, scallions, garlic, ginger, water chestnuts, soy sauce, ketchup, white wine, and cayenne pepper

FRIED RICE, YANG CHOW with rice, black mushrooms, ginger, shrimp, ham, water chestnuts, peas, soy sauce, egg, scallions, and romaine lettuce

LO MEIN, PORK with pork, Chinese mushrooms, cornstarch, wheat-flour noodles, ginger, scallions, bamboo shoots, zucchini, soy sauce, oyster sauce, and sesame oil

LO MEIN, VEGETABLE with Chinese mushrooms, wheat-flour noodles, vegetable stock, oyster sauce, celery, bamboo shoots, bean sprouts, and scallions

RICE STICK NOODLES WITH SINGAPORE-STYLE SHRIMP with rice noodles, shrimp, garlic, onion, curry powder, coconut milk, and cayenne

Salads
Lowest Fat: *Shredded Cucumber and Bean Threads with Drunken Shrimp—16.8 g fat, 344.8 calories*
Highest Fat: *Hoisin Beef Salad—34 g fat, 455.5 calories*

HOISIN BEEF SALAD with beef, plum sauce, red potatoes, lettuce, mustard, lime juice, soy sauce, sesame oil, olive oil, and red onion

SHREDDED CUCUMBER AND BEAN THREADS WITH DRUNKEN SHRIMP with cucumber, bean threads, shrimp, horseradish, mustard, garlic, soy sauce, olive oil, vegetable oil, chives, sherry, ginger, and brandy

Desserts
Lowest Fat: *Lichee Sorbet—0 g fat, 53 calories*
Highest Fat: *Star Anise Rice Pudding—17 g fat, 439 calories*

ALMOND COOKIES *Hsing Jen Ping* with lard, almond extract, and slivered almonds

Serving Size	Calories	Fat (g)	Sodium (mg)	Carbohydrate (g)	Cholesterol (mg)	Fiber (g)
1½ cups	432.9	19	**1304.1**	45.7	270.5	0.4
1½ cups	423	17.4	**1147.5**	48	241.5	0.7
1½ cups	778	33	**1070**	82.8	63.7	0.5
1½ cups	543	13	610	85.4	1.9	1.1
1½ cups	573	10	690	88.1	173.3	0.4
1 cup	455.5	34	329	16	78.3	0.7
1 cup	344.8	16.8	876	6.6	184.9	0.4
1 cookie	59	4	22	6	7.8	.02

CHINESE DISHES

FOOD NAME

FORTUNE COOKIES   with egg, flour, and confectioners' sugar
ORANGE WEDGES   oranges
LICHEE SORBET
SESAME PUFFS WITH HONEY   deep-fried in vegetable oil
STAR ANISE RICE PUDDING   made with milk, heavy cream, sugar, and egg yolks
SWEET CRESCENTS   with sesame seeds, chopped dates, currants, dried apricots, peanut butter, and brown sugar in wonton skins, deep-fried in vegetable oil

Serving Size	Calories	Fat (g)	Sodium (mg)	Carbohydrate (g)	Cholesterol (mg)	Fiber (g)
1 cookie	82.75	5.2	0.2	8.35	0	.04
1 orange	65	0.2	1	5.41	0	4
½ cup	53	0	0	14.2	0	0.2
1 small puff	88.3	5.2	20	8.8	28.8	.04
¾ cup	**439**	**17**	34	67.4	248.9	0.1
1 crescent	68	4	6.1	7.6	0	0.2

French Cuisine

Traditionally a very rich, cream-intensive cuisine, French cooking can be a minefield for the unwary diner, and presents a special challenge for patrons seeking low-fat meals. Still, there are always healthy alternatives to fat-saturated choices. Look for items that are steamed, roasted, poached, puréed, *en brochette* (grilled), *en papillote* (in parchment or foil), or prepared with wine and herbs. Foods designated *au beurre, au gratin, hollandaise, béchamel, mayonnaise, mornay,* and *crème* contain large amounts of butter, cream and/or cheese, all of which are high in fat. Fruit-based sauces contain no fat and should be elected over cream-based ones. If you're unsure about the sauce, ask for it to be served on the side. A good rule of thumb is that any savory sauce too thick to see through is probably high in fat. Rather than a meal centered on red meat, stick to fish and poultry, and order a good dose of fresh or steamed vegetables (skip the butter). Traditional French desserts are monuments to the use of lard and cream. Wait until you get home to eat dessert, or order a fruit dessert (minus the whipped cream) and coffee.

FRENCH DISHES

FOOD NAME
Soups and Appetizers *Lowest Fat:* Tuna Mousse—3.5 g fat, 64 calories *Highest Fat:* Puff Pastry with Anchovy Butter—30.2 g fat, 341.3 calories
CHICKEN LIVER MOUSSE *Mousse de Foie de Volaille* with chicken livers, shallots, Madeira, and Cognac
CREAM OF ASPARAGUS SOUP *Crème d'Asperges* with asparagus, chicken stock and heavy cream
ESCARGOTS snails served in shells with consommé, white wine, and butter flavored with shallots, garlic, and parsley
FRENCH ONION SOUP *Soupe à l'Oignon Gratinée* made with beef stock, onion, Cognac, and Swiss-style cheese
HOME-STYLE PÂTÉ WITH PRUNES *Terrine Maison aux Pruneaux* with ham, chicken, white wine, Cognac, Madeira, pork fat, pork, and veal
MEDITERRANEAN FISH SOUP *Soupe de Poisson* made with skinless fish fillets, fish stock, fennel, onion, tomatoes, saffron, garlic, orange zest, and white wine
PUFF PASTRY WITH ANCHOVY BUTTER *Feuilletés d'Anchois* hors d'oeuvres made with anchovy fillets, butter, lemon, and Dijon mustard
TUNA MOUSSE with prunes, onion, parsley, light cream cheese, ricotta cheese, white tuna, pecans, and lemon juice
VICHYSOISSE leek and potato soup with consommé, milk, and butter

Serving Size	Calories	Fat (g)	Sodium (mg)	Carbohydrate (g)	Cholesterol (mg)	Fiber (g)
2 oz	230	20.3	293.8	1.3	287.2	0.1
1¼ cups	**854.4**	5.2	545.6	5.3	13.4	0.6
6 snails	193.4	17.7	517.4	1.4	85.6	0.1
1½ cups	333.1	21.3	**1187.5**	14.5	65.5	0.3
2 oz	159.8	10.5	180	3.7	47.4	.13
1¾ cups	292.2	16.5	170.2	12.6	37.5	1.1
6 small pastries	341.3	**30.2**	**400.1**	9.2	102.8	0.1
1½ oz	64	3.5	120	1.6	11	0.3
1 cup	317.9	13.9	747	40.2	37.2	1.5

FRENCH DISHES

FOOD NAME

Meat Dishes

Lowest Fat: Braised Artichokes with Ham and Vegetables—13.6 g fat, 305.3 calories

Highest Fat: Roasted Fillet of Beef—107.3 g fat, 1259.3 calories

---

BRAISED ARTICHOKES WITH HAM AND VEGETABLES *Artichauts Barigoule* with artichokes, ham, olive oil, onions, carrots, celery, garlic, white wine, and beef stock

BRAISED BRISKET WITH GINGER AND CORIANDER *Poitrine de Boeuf Braisée au Gingembre et Coriandre* with beef, onions, carrots, garlic, shallots, red wine, beef stock, tomato paste, and new potatoes

BURGUNDY-STYLE BEEF STEW *Boeuf Bourguignon* with beef chuck, onions, carrots, Cognac, red wine, beef stock, garlic, tomato paste, pearl onions, new potatoes, bacon, and mushrooms

FILET MIGNON panfried steak with bacon, butter, oil, salt and pepper

FILLET STEAKS WITH MUSHROOMS AND BÉARNAISE SAUCE *Tournedos Charlemagne* fillet steaks with butter, shallots, mushrooms, tomato paste, white wine, and egg yolks

FRENCH LAMB STEW *Navarin d'Agneau* lamb with beef stock, white wine, tomato paste, garlic, carrots, pearl onions, turnips, and new potatoes

GRILLED RIB STEAK *Côte de Boeuf Grillée* steak with watercress

HAM AND MUSHROOM CRÊPES WITH CHEESE SAUCE *Crêpes au Jambon Sauce Mornay* with ham, mushrooms, and Gruyère cheese

ONE-POT MEAL WITH CHICKEN, PORK, SAUSAGE AND VEGETABLES *Potée* with chicken, pork, sausage, carrots, onions, cloves, garlic, celery, turnips, cabbage, and potatoes

Serving Size	Calories	Fat (g)	Sodium (mg)	Carbohydrate (g)	Cholesterol (mg)	Fiber (g)
1 medium artichoke	305.3	13.6	864.5	28.1	16.2	1.4
12 oz	699.7	40.1	458	33.8	122.5	1.03
1½ cups	691.0	43.4	709.7	26.1	142.3	1.9
8 oz	661.6	53.1	377.4	0.0	178.9	0.0
1 8-oz fillet	**1088.4**	**99.4**	**800.4**	5.2	402.5	1.2
12 oz	781.5	48.3	602.1	46.8	112.5	1.64
8 oz	753.3	66.0	213.8	0.3	163	0.1
2 crêpes, each with ¾ oz filling	510.7	42.7	745.6	15.5	205	0.8
1¼ cups broth and 12 oz meat and vegetables	858.5	53.8	**1012.4**	26.6	243.9	1.4

FRENCH DISHES

FOOD NAME

PEPPER-COATED STEAK WITH COGNAC AND CREAM *Steak au Poivre* Steak with Cognac, pepper, and cream, served on a bed of watercress

PORK MEDALLIONS WITH A MUSTARD BROWN SAUCE *Medaillons de Porc Sauce Robert* pork with butter, Cognac, white wine, Dijon mustard, and parsley

RACK OF LAMB *Carré d'Agneau Vert Pré* lamb with thyme, rosemary, and watercress

ROAST LEG OF LAMB *Gigot d'Agneau Rôti* lamb with garlic, thyme, and rosemary

ROAST PORK WITH PRUNES *Rôti de Porc aux Pruneaux* pork with thyme, onions, carrots, butter, white raisins, red wine, beef stock, and port

ROASTED FILLET OF BEEF *Filet de Boeuf Rôti* beef with butter, carrots, onions, beef stock, and béarnaise sauce

SAUTÉED RABBIT WITH MUSTARD AND ROSEMARY SAUCE *Lapin Sauté à la Moutarde et au Romarin* rabbit with onions, garlic, shallots, mustard, Cognac, white wine, chicken stock, rosemary, and heavy cream

SAUTÉED VEAL SCALLOPS WITH MUSHROOMS AND TOMATO SAUCE *Escalopes de Veau Chasseur* veal scallops with white wine, beef stock, tomato paste, and Cognac

VEAL PRINCE ORLOFF roast veal with bacon, onions, rice, heavy cream, flour, butter, Gruyère and Parmesan cheese

VEAL STEW WITH WILD MUSHROOMS *Blanquette de Veau aux Morilles* Veal with onions, carrots, leeks, turnips, celery, pearl onions, butter, egg yolks, and heavy cream

Serving Size	Calories	Fat (g)	Sodium (mg)	Carbohydrate (g)	Cholesterol (mg)	Fiber (g)
1 10-oz steak	984.1	79.5	301.6	1.7	246.6	.13
1 8-oz medallion	434.7	31.9	363.4	4.3	88.8	.14
12 oz (½ rack)	918.9	77.6	290.4	0.3	216.0	0.1
10 oz	1070	74.2	321.3	0.3	309.2	.02
12 oz	1610	41.4	420.2	33.9	171.3	1.4
10 oz	**1259.3**	**107.3**	633.6	20	**372.0**	0.2
12 oz	610.5	38.8	360.2	4.9	226.6	.25
8 oz	277.5	19.1	386.6	3.1	86.8	0.7
12 oz	797.4	60.1	**1323.9**	26.1	198	0.3
1½ cups	525.2	31.7	305.7	17.4	245.2	1.4

FRENCH DISHES

FOOD NAME

Poultry Dishes

Lowest Fat: Cornish Hens with Herbs and Mustard—10.5 g fat, 398 calories

Highest Fat: Duck with Orange Sauce—185.8 g fat, 2057.8 calories

CHICKEN IN A POT *Poule au Pot* chicken with chicken stock, leeks, onions, turnips, carrots, celery, and rice

CHICKEN IN RED WINE *Coq au Vin* chicken with onions, shallots, garlic, beef stock, tomato paste, pearl onions, bacon, and mushrooms

CHICKEN SAUTÉED WITH HAM, PEPPERS AND TOMATOES *Suprêmes de Volaille Basquaise* chicken breast meat, onions, prosciutto, garlic, red and green peppers, and butter

CHICKEN STUFFED WITH TRUFFLES *Poularde Truffée et Farcie* chicken roasted, with truffles, smoked bacon, onions, chicken livers, bread crumbs, Madeira, butter, and carrots

CHICKEN WITH CREAMY TARRAGON SAUCE *Poularde Pochée à l'Estragon* chicken poached, with chicken stock, carrot, onions, butter, flour, and heavy cream

CHICKEN WITH MUSHROOMS, TOMATOES, AND OLIVES *Poulet Sauté à la Portugaise* chicken with mushrooms, tomatoes, green and black olives, butter, onions, garlic, shallots, beef stock, white wine, and parsley

CHICKEN WITH SHERRY VINEGAR *Poulet au Vinaigre de Xérès* chicken with butter, onions, shallots, garlic, white wine, tomato paste, and parsley

CORNISH HENS WITH HERBS AND MUSTARD *Poussins aux Herbes et à la Moutarde* broiled cornish hens with Dijon mustard, tarragon, basil, thyme, and white wine

Serving Size	Calories	Fat (g)	Sodium (mg)	Carbohydrate (g)	Cholesterol (mg)	Fiber (g)
2 cups	887.1	40.1	**1968.8**	23.8	247	1.2
2 cups	**1102.6**	69	942	11.3	324.6	0.9
12 oz	527.8	22.2	637.5	17.2	187.3	1.9
10 oz	**1040.8**	64.3	835.5	8.6	603	0.2
10 oz	683.1	39.5	**1485**	5.1	265	0.1
2 cups	937.2	51.3	**1042.3**	20.3	318.8	2.6
6 oz	655.9	37.3	465.8	6.6	251.5	0.3
12 oz (½ hen)	398	10.5	275.1	1.7	179.2	0.2

FRENCH DISHES

FOOD NAME

DUCK WITH ORANGE SAUCE *Canard à l'Orange* duck with onion, carrot, fresh oranges and orange zest, white wine, beef stock, garlic, tomato paste, Madeira, and Cognac

PHEASANT WITH JUNIPER *Suprêmes de Faisan au Genévrier* Pheasant with fresh juniper berries, butter, gin, and heavy cream

DUCK, ROASTED *Canard Rôti* duck roasted, with onion, carrot, celery, shallots, parsley, and chicken stock

SQUABS WITH OLIVE SAUCE *Pigeonneaux aux Olives* squab with olive oil, onion, carrot, white wine, beef stock, tomato paste, and green olives

Fish and Shellfish Dishes
Lowest Fat: Baked Snapper in a Mediterranean Tomato Sauce— 6.4 g fat, 419.5 calories
Highest Fat: Strips of Fried Sole, Fried Parsley, and Onion Rings— 106.5 g fat, 1187.1 calories

BAKED SNAPPER IN A MEDITERRANEAN TOMATO SAUCE *Rouget à la Méditerranée* snapper with olive oil, onion, shallots, cloves, fennel, saffron and parsley

FISH MOUSSELINE *Mousseline de Poisson* with boneless fish, shrimp, egg whites, nutmeg, and heavy cream

MEDITERRANEAN FISH STEW *Bouillabaise* with onion, leek, fennel, garlic, tomato, lobster, mussels, fish fillets, shrimp, sea scallops, French bread, aïoli, and rouille

MONKFISH IN A SPICY TOMATO SAUCE *Lotte à l'Americaine* with olive oil, onion, shallots, garlic, Cognac, white wine, tarragon, tomato paste, and fresh tomatoes

SALMON FILLETS WITH BUTTER SAUCE *Filet de Saumon Poché Sauce Beurre Blanc* poached salmon fillets with Beurre Blanc

Serving Size	Calories	Fat (g)	Sodium (mg)	Carbohydrate (g)	Cholesterol (mg)	Fiber (g)
13 oz	**2057.8**	**185.8**	645.2	28.8	348.8	0.8
10 oz	494.7	23.7	283.4	1.4	215.4	0
13 oz	**1881.6**	**181.4**	736.9	3.5	349.1	0.3
1 medium squab	555	35.7	983.1	10.7	182	0.9
10 oz	419.5	6.4	424.2	15.3	124	1.7
7 oz	324.1	24.2	392.2	2.7	189.5	0
2½ cups	941.7	40.6	**1561.8**	32.5	476.3	0.5
2 cups	362.4	14.6	190.6	13.4	66.3	1.3
8 oz	601	45	411.3	3.1	208	0.1

FRENCH DISHES

FOOD NAME

SALMON, POACHED, WITH GREEN MAYONNAISE *Saumon Poché Sauce Verte* poached salmon steaks served cold with shallots, vinegar, lemon, parsley, watercress, tarragon, chervil, basil, and egg

SHRIMP AND SCALLOPS IN PUFF-PASTRY SHELLS *Bouchées de Fruits de Mer* with shrimp, scallops, shallots, mushrooms, white wine, egg yolks, and butter

SHRIMP IN A GARLIC TOMATO SAUCE *Crevettes à la Provençale* Shrimp with olive oil, fresh tomatoes, and parsley

SOLE, FRIED PARSLEY, AND ONION RINGS *Goujonnettes de Sole* deep-fried strips of sole served with lemon and rémoulade sauce

SOLE WITH SHRIMP, MUSHROOMS, AND TRUFFLES *Filet de Sole Granville* filet with butter, fish stock, egg yolks, heavy cream, and white wine

Organ Meats

BRAISED STUFFED HEART with beef heart, beef broth, flour, onion, carrot, celery, rice and parsley

CHICKEN LIVERS WITH VINEGAR AND ONIONS *Foies de Volaille au Vinaigre de Vin et aux Oignons* chicken livers with milk, butter, anchovies, sugar, flour, and chicken stock, served with French bread

SAUTÉED BRAINS with flour, salt, pepper, butter and toast

SAUTÉED CALF"S LIVER with butter, nutmeg, savory, salt and pepper

Sauces
Lowest Fat: *Crème Anglais*—12.4 g fat, 285.5 calories
Highest Fat: *Béarnaise Sauce*—29.9 g fat, 270.6 calories

BÉCHAMEL with milk, flour, butter, nutmeg, and onion flavor

Serving Size	Calories	Fat (g)	Sodium (mg)	Carbohydrate (g)	Cholesterol (mg)	Fiber (g)
8 oz	777.1	62.7	**2850**	5.8	203.3	0.5
1 8-oz pastry	594.1	41.6	**7650**	16.3	340.9	.44
1½ cups	278.9	13.6	325.2	10	208	0.9
10 oz	**1187.1**	**106.5**	574.2	19.7	88.3	0.4
10 oz	462.8	22.4	879.8	5.9	329	0.6
10 oz	534.7	20.1	835.5	19.8	434.0	.26
4 oz	600.9	29.9	**1072.8**	38.8	**749.1**	0.4
5 oz	349.5	25.1	897.2	14.6	**1951.0**	.02
6 oz	339.1	19.5	507.6	7.0	541.4	0
⅓ cup	182.5	13.1	424.6	10.9	42.7	0

FRENCH DISHES

FOOD NAME

BÉARNAISE SAUCE with butter, egg yolks, white wine, tarragon, shallots, chervil, and tarragon vinegar

CRÈME ANGLAIS with whole milk, eggs, and sugar

HOLLANDAISE with butter, lemon juice, and egg yolks

MORNAY with flour, butter, milk, and onions

Casseroles, Soufflés, Noodles, and Omelets
Lowest Fat: Spinach Soufflé—16.5 g fat, 278.9 calories
Highest Fat: White Bean Casserole with Duck, Pork, Lamb, and Sausage—187.4 g fat, 2159.5 calories

NOODLES WITH CREAM, PEAS, AND PARMESAN *Pâtes Fraîches aux Petits Pois* noodles with heavy cream, ham, peas, and parmesan cheese

OMELET, HERB *Omelette aux Fine Herbes* with 3 eggs, chives, tarragon, parsley, and butter

QUICHE LORRAINE with flour, salt, butter, mustard, eggs, bacon, whole milk, nutmeg, and Gruyère cheese

QUICHE, ONION with eggs, onions, red peppers, mushrooms, Monterey Jack cheese, and sour cream in pie crust

SOUFFLÉ, HAM *Soufflé au Jambon* with eggs, ham, whole milk, Madeira, and mustard

SOUFFLÉ, ROQUEFORT CHEESE *Soufflé au Roquefort* with eggs, cheese, whole milk, Dijon mustard, and nutmeg

SOUFFLÉ, SPINACH *Soufflé aux Épinards* with eggs, whole milk, spinach, and nutmeg

ONION TART *Tarte à l'Oignon* made with pâte brisée, onion, butter, eggs, whole milk and nutmeg

Serving Size	Calories	Fat (g)	Sodium (mg)	Carbohydrate (g)	Cholesterol (mg)	Fiber (g)
¼ cup	270.6	**29.9**	390.8	0.9	183.2	0.03
½ cup	285.5	12.4	163.5	30.4	427.5	0
¼ cup	250.4	27.2	374.4	0.4	266	0
¼ cup	163.2	13	291.4	4.6	91.9	0.1
11 oz	363.8	19.9	402.9	35.2	67.1	0.7
1 6-oz omelet	305.1	17.7	607	11.5	314.3	0.1
6 oz	389.5	25.7	600.4	160	225.8	0.2
6 oz	519	33.8	**1452**	41.4	174	0.5
9 oz	389.1	25.1	698.3	11.7	**679.6**	0.1
8 oz	341.6	22.2	490.5	13.7	321	0.1
8 oz	278.9	16.5	507.1	14.7	303.7	0.3
6 oz	313.1	20.3	322.2	16.9	203.2	0.2

FRENCH DISHES

FOOD NAME

WHITE BEAN CASSEROLE WITH DUCK, PORK, LAMB, AND SAUSAGE *Cassoulet* with duck, pork, lamb, sausage, white wine, and white beans

French—Vegetables
Lowest Fat: *Potatoes and Onions Baked in Stock—2.8 g fat, 265 calories*
Highest Fat: *French-fried Potatoes—78 g fat, 870 calories*

BROILED TOMATOES WITH GARLIC AND HERBS *Tomates à la Provençale* broiled tomatoes, with bread crumbs, thyme, olive oil, and parsley

CAULIFLOWER PURÉE *Purée de Choux-fleurs* with cauliflower, potatoes, whole milk, and butter

LEEKS IN CREAM *Poireaux à la Crème* leeks with butter and heavy cream

MUSHROOM STUFFING WITH SHALLOTS *Duxelles* with mushrooms, shallots, butter, salt, and pepper

MUSHROOMS AND GARLIC *Champignons à l'Ail* mushrooms sautéed in butter and garlic

MUSHROOMS IN CREAM SAUCE *Champignons à la Créme* with mushrooms, butter, shallots, heavy cream, and dry sherry

MUSHROOMS, MARINATED *Champignons à la Grecque* mushrooms with white wine, olive oil, lemon, shallots, garlic, and tomatoes

POTATOES WITH GARLIC, MASHED *Purée de Pommes de Terre à l'Ail* with potatoes, garlic, salt and freshly ground pepper

POTATOES AND ONIONS BAKED IN STOCK *Pommes de Terre à la Boulangere* potatoes with butter, salt, pepper, and chicken stock

POTATOES, FRENCH-FRIED *Pommes Frites* potatoes fried in oil

POTATOES, SAUTÉED *Pommes de Terre Sautées* with butter and parsley

Serving Size	Calories	Fat (g)	Sodium (mg)	Carbohydrate (g)	Cholesterol (mg)	Fiber (g)
2 cups	**2159.5**	**187.4**	**1644**	31.7	**426.5**	2.2
5 oz	82.6	7	64.6	4.8	0	0.4
1¼ cups	114.3	6.3	300.3	14	15.6	0.9
6 oz	144.9	7.9	**1260**	17.9	24.3	1.9
⅓ cup	67.8	5.9	193.9	3.6	15.5	1.2
¾ cup	60	5.7	129.3	2.2	13.3	0.9
⅔ cup	145.5	14.3	122.9	30	49.3	0.7
5 oz	139.4	11.1	434.6	6.1	0	1.6
1¼ cups	295	1.3	345.4	64.3	3.3	1.7
1¼ cups	265	2.8	644	53.3	5.5	1.4
10 oz	**870**	**78**	118.6	25.7	0	1.6
8 oz	239.2	8	175.2	38.7	20.7	1

FRENCH DISHES

FOOD NAME

POTATOES ROASTED WITH BUTTER *Pommes de Terre Rôties*

POTATOES SLICED AND BAKED IN CREAM *Gratin Dauphinois* with potatoes, garlic, whole milk, and heavy cream

POTATO PUFFS *Pommes de Terre Dauphiné* mashed potatoes mixed with cream-puff pastry, deep-fried in vegetable oil

RATATOUILLE NIÇOISE with olive oil, onions, green peppers, garlic, zucchini, eggplant, tomatoes, and tomato paste

SPINACH, CREAMED *Purée d'Épinards* with nutmeg and Béchamel Sauce

WHITE BEANS WITH GARLIC AND TOMATOES *Haricots à la Bretonne* with carrots, onions, butter, and parsley

Desserts
Lowest Fat: *Chocolate-Almond Macaroon—2.6 g fat, 36.6 calories*
Highest Fat: *Napoleon—104.3 g fat, 1443.9 calories*

ALMOND CAKE WITH A RASPBERRY PURÉE *Pain de Genes sur Coulis de Framboise* with Kirsch liqueur, sugar, butter, flour, eggs, vanilla, and dark rum

ALMOND MERINGUE AND BUTTERCREAM LAYER CAKE *Gâteau aux Fonds à Succès* with butter, almonds, sugar, cornstarch, eggs, and flavored syrup

ALMOND TILE COOKIES *Tuiles aux Amandes* with butter, egg whites, vanilla, and blanched almonds

ALSATIAN FRUIT TART *Tarte Alsacienne aux Fruits* with almonds, sugar, egg yolks, milk, vanilla, apples, apricots, cherries, pears, and plums, and apricot glaze

APRICOT JAM ROLL *Biscuit Roulé à l'Abricot* with eggs, sugar, orange juice, flour, butter, apricot jam, and almonds

BANANAS FLAMBÉED IN RUM *Bananes Flambées au Rhum* with bananas, sugar, butter, lemon juice, dark rum, and almonds

Serving Size	Calories	Fat (g)	Sodium (mg)	Carbohydrate (g)	Cholesterol (mg)	Fiber (g)
8 oz	272	11.8	213.3	38.6	31	1
10 oz	403.8	17.9	438.2	54.6	60	1.3
6 oz	614.5	55	444.3	22.3	134.4	0.5
1¾ cups	174.3	9.7	106.5	220	0	2.2
½ cup	170.8	11.1	556.6	110	36.1	0.2
1 cup	155.5	5.8	162.9	21.3	14.1	1.6
4 oz	465.5	23.8	178.6	56.5	118.1	0.4
4 oz	493.2	39.1	271.4	32.6	315.5	0.5
2 cookies	178.2	13.2	66.4	11.8	64	0.4
6 oz	439.3	17.1	139.6	64.4	184.9	1
5 oz	406.8	11.1	91.1	67.4	193	0.5
5 oz	387.3	16.9	119.1	43.6	310	0.8

FRENCH DISHES

FOOD NAME

BLUEBERRY TART *Tarte aux Myrtilles* with fresh blueberries, sugar, and currant jelly glaze in pastry crust
CARAMEL CUSTARD *Crème Caramel* with milk, sugar, eggs, and vanilla
CHOCOLATE-ALMOND MACAROONS *Macarons au Chocolat* egg whites and cocoa powder
CHOCOLATE-COATED HAZELNUT AND ALMOND COOKIES *Biarritz* with sugar, butter, egg whites, flour, chocolate, vanilla, hazelnuts and almonds
CHOCOLATE GÉNOISE WITH APRICOT GLAZE AND CHOCOLATE ICING with eggs, butter, sugar, flour, cocoa, raspberry jam, orange juice, and apricot glaze
CHOCOLATE MOUSSE *Mousse au Chocolat* with semisweet chocolate, butter, and eggs
CHOCOLATE MOUSSE CAKE *Gâteau Mousse au Chocolat* with cocoa powder, chocolate, butter, and eggs
COINTREAU OMELET *Omelette au Cointreau* made with eggs, sugar, and butter
CRÊPES SUZETTE with flour, eggs, vanilla, milk, butter, sugar, orange juice and zest, and Grand Marnier
FLOATING ISLAND WITH RASPBERRY SAUCE *Île Flottante* with egg whites, sugar, vanilla, almonds, crème anglaise, and coulis de framboise
MADELEINES with butter, eggs, lemon zest, and flour
NAPOLEONS *Mille-feuilles* with puff pastry, pastry cream, and Grand Marnier

Serving Size	Calories	Fat (g)	Sodium (mg)	Carbohydrate (g)	Cholesterol (mg)	Fiber (g)
4 oz	357.6	120	133.2	58.9	104.9	1.1
5 oz	207.6	7.7	85.6	29.2	196.7	0
3 cookies	109.8	7.8	9.3	9.6	34.2	0.4
3 cookies	147.9	11.4	54.6	11.4	37.5	0.2
1 3-oz piece	411.0	25.5	40	45.6	146.8	0.4
2 oz	216	18.1	124.7	11.2	203.3	0.2
3 oz	375.8	31.6	134.4	13.8	**655.4**	0.2
2 oz	262.6	11.2	133.6	21.4	418.8	0
3 6-inch crêpes	375.9	22.6	240	27.1	173.2	0.1
5 oz	392.4	15	106.8	59.7	288.8	0.2
2 madeleines	157.2	9.2	95.8	13.6	89.2	.04
5 oz	**1443.9**	**104.3**	**1537.6**	75.4	**535.8**	0.5

FRENCH DISHES

FOOD NAME

ORANGE-CHOCOLATE GÉNOISE WITH GRAND MARNIER–CHOCOLATE ICING *Gâteau Chocolat au Grand Marnier* with flour, sugar, eggs, butter, cocoa, orange juice, heavy cream, and semisweet chocolate

PUFF PASTRY WITH STRAWBERRIES *Feuilleté aux Fraises* with currant jelly, Kirsch liqueur, and almonds

RUM CAKE *Savarin au Rhum* with butter, flour, eggs, vanilla, rum, sugar, apricot glaze, and almonds

SOUFFLÉ, APRICOT *Soufflé à l'Abricot* with egg whites, dried apricots, and orange liqueur

SOUFFLÉ, CHOCOLATE, WITH GRAND MARNIER *Soufflé au Chocolat et au Grand Marnier* with eggs, butter, semisweet chocolate, orange zest, and Grand Marnier

SOUFFLÉ, GRAND MARNIER *Soufflé au Grand Marnier* with milk, eggs, butter, sugar, orange, and Grand Marnier

SOUFFLÉ, ORANGE OMELET *Orange Omelette Soufflé* with eggs, sugar, orange zest, and confectioners' sugar

UPSIDE-DOWN CARAMELIZED APPLE TART *Tarte Tatin* with butter, sugar, lemon juice, and apples in tart pastry

VANILLA AND COFFEE CUSTARDS *Pots de Crème: Vanille et Cafe* with light cream, sugar, eggs, vanilla, and instant coffee

VANILLA GÉNOISE WITH COFFEE BUTTERCREAM *Gâteau Moka* with sugar, coffee, almonds, egg yolks, butter, and flour

Serving Size	Calories	Fat (g)	Sodium (mg)	Carbohydrate (g)	Cholesterol (mg)	Fiber (g)
2½ oz	330	20.6	75.6	31.1	146.8	0.4
6 oz	291.8	6.1	17.1	55.6	34.3	0.9
4 oz	300.1	9.4	86.9	38.7	85.9	0.1
5 oz	301.4	12.8	145.3	36.3	358	0.2
3 oz	463.3	330	245.9	36.2	320.5	0.3
5 oz	327.4	12.1	95.8	38.7	227.8	.04
4 oz	319.6	9.6	118.6	48.2	**469.8**	0
8 oz	440	26.2	**1940**	49.2	92.9	1.4
⅔ cup	240.6	10.8	90.2	27.8	335.3	0
3 oz	428	30.7	231.7	30.4	268.6	0.3

German and Austrian Cuisine

Americans tend to think of German or Austrian cuisine as "comfort food." Heavy on the meat and potatoes, these stick-to-the-ribs dishes are the perfect choice for a cold fall or winter day; however, this cuisine is rarely the best choice for a serious dieter since many dishes are laden with heavy sauces and fatty meats. One way to enjoy these delicacies is to order half portions and eat in moderation. Another strategy is to choose two side dishes—perhaps a steamed vegetable or a dish of sauerkraut along with a simple potato dish in place of a meat entree. When that Schnitzel is just too good to pass up, your best choices for meat dishes are meats that are roasted (without the skin), grilled, or boiled. Ask for the sauces to be served on the side and share that delicious dessert with the rest of the table. German and Austrian pastries are famous around the world.

GERMAN AND AUSTRIAN DISHES

FOOD NAME

Soups and Beverages
Lowest Fat: Cabbage Soup—13.6 g fat-153 calories
Highest Fat: Potato Soup—14.6 g fat, 195.9 calories

PEACH BOWL *Pfirsichbowle* with peaches, powdered sugar, sherry, and dry white wine

CABBAGE SOUP with onion, butter, cabbage, beef broth, grated cheese, and sour cream

SPICED WINE *Glühwein* spiced red wine with sugar, lemon, and cloves

POTATO SOUP *Kartoffelsuppe* with onion, butter, chicken broth, potato, celery salt, milk, cream, white pepper, and parsley

Side Dishes
Lowest Fat: Stuffed Onions—0.5 g fat, 46.8 calories
Highest Fat: Spatzle—25.7 g fat, 454 calories

BRUSSELS SPROUTS with brussels sprouts, butter, grated Parmesan cheese, chopped parsley, lemon juice, and nutmeg

CABBAGE, STUFFED *Gefüllter Krautkopf* with cabbage, bread, ham, pork, onion, egg, milk, pepper, herbs, and butter

DUMPLINGS *Nockerl* with butter, egg, flour, salt, and milk

DUMPLINGS, LIVER *Leberklösse* or *Leberknödel* with liver, egg, bread crumbs, cream, marjoram, parsley, onion, garlic and butter

MEAT PÂTÉ *Leberkäse* with pork, butter, and onions

ONIONS, STUFFED with onions, sauerkraut, bread crumbs and caraway seeds

POTATO SALAD *Kartoffelsalat, Warmer* hot, with potatoes, bacon, onion, celery, dill pickle, vinegar, sugar, salt, and paprika

SAUERKRAUT with cabbage, butter, onion, potato, and caraway seeds

SPATZLE with flour, egg, butter, and spices

Serving Size	Calories	Fat (g)	Sodium (mg)	Carbohydrate (g)	Cholesterol (mg)	Fiber (g)
1 cup	296.2	0	14.4	32.4	0	0.2
1 cup	153	13.6	**912.2**	3.4	35.4	0.2
1 cup	265.3	0	22.8	29.5	0	0
1 cup	**195.9**	14.6	815.8	12.3	48.8	0.3
⅔ cup	67	3.4	113.5	6.7	8.3	1.1
2 3-oz rolls	354.3	**22.2**	**1150.7**	10.6	181.9	0.3
1 oz	352.4	18.8	280.8	23.2	136	0.2
1¼ oz	43.9	2.7	171.1	2.2	56.5	0
1 oz	195	17	471	6.5	48	0.4
1 5-oz onion	46.8	0.5	554.0	9.8	0	0.9
¾ cup	110.1	2.3	491.1	20.1	3.6	0.6
¾ cup	85.2	4.2	**1080.4**	12	10.3	1.9
½ cup	**454**	**25.7**	680	43	170.2	0.2

GERMAN AND AUSTRIAN DISHES

FOOD NAME

Sausages, Wieners, and Wursts
Lowest Fat: Bierwurst—21.6 g fat, 268 calories
Highest Fat: Bauernwurst—34.2 g fat, 354 calories

BAUERNWURST   highly seasoned and coarsely textured sausage

BIERWURST   soft, cooked sausage

BRATWURST   with veal, pork, caraway seeds, lemon, and ginger

KNOCKWURST   short, chunky frankfurter, highly seasoned with garlic

LIVERWURST   smooth-textured liver pâté in casing

WEISSWURST   with veal, cream, and eggs

WIENERS   with beef and/or pork

Main Dishes
Lowest Fat: Pork Chops with Sauerkraut—14.9 g fat, 256.7 calories
Highest Fat: Sauerbraten—66.3 g fat, 867.8 calories

BEEF BRISKET WITH SAUERKRAUT   *Gedämpfte Rinderbrust mit Sauerkraut*   beef with bacon fat, onions, apple, salt, and pepper

BOILED BEEF   *Gekochtes Rindfleisch*   with beef, onion, carrots, celery, salt, turnip, butter, cloves, and horseradish

PORK CHOPS WITH SAUERKRAUT   *Schweinekotelette mit Sauerkraut*   pork chops with bacon, applesauce, brown sugar, white wine, mustard, and ground pepper

RABBIT STEW   *Hasenpfeffer*   with rabbit, peppercorns, mustard seed, cloves, cider vinegar, onion, flour, dry red wine, and butter

BRAISED BEEF ROLLS   *Rouladen*   with beef, flour, oil, celery, mushrooms, broth, capers, onions, and bacon

MARINATED POT ROAST   *Sauerbraten*   with beef shoulder, vinegar, onions, peppercorns, caraway seeds, sugar, cream, and flour

Serving Size	Calories	Fat (g)	Sodium (mg)	Carbohydrate (g)	Cholesterol (mg)	Fiber (g)
1 3-oz link	354	**34.2**	567	0.9	57	0
1 4-oz link	268	21.6	**1408**	2.4	68	0
1 4-oz link	341.2	29.2	630.8	2.4	68	0
1 4-oz link	278.8	25.2	**916**	1.6	52	0
1 oz	93	8.1	250	0.6	45	0
1 2-oz link	174	15.6	300	0.2	68	0
1 oz	96	8.7	336	0.8	14.7	0
10 oz	561.8	37.6	**1634**	10.8	147	1.9
8 oz	550.4	38.5	553.2	4.8	167.7	0.4
1 5-oz chop	256.7	14.9	812.8	21.2	40.5	2
6 oz	416.6	22.5	155.6	8.2	168.2	0.1
6 oz	423.1	22.6	**1145**	5.8	115.8	0.4
8 oz	**867.8**	**66.3**	332.6	25	209.8	0.1

GERMAN AND AUSTRIAN DISHES

FOOD NAME

SCHNITZEL, CREAM *Rahmschnitzel* veal cutlet coated with flour, fried, and covered with beef broth, light cream, and sour cream

SCHNITZEL, PAPRIKA veal cutlet coated in flour and paprika, fried, and covered with beef broth and sour cream

SCHNITZEL, PLAIN *Naturschnitzel* veal cutlet coated in flour, salt, and pepper, and then fried

SCHNITZEL, WEINER *Weinerschnitzel* veal cutlet coated with egg, bread crumbs, and milk, then fried in butter

VEAL PAPRIKASH with veal shoulder, butter, onions, garlic, paprika, white wine, tomato, and sour cream

Desserts
Lowest Fat: Pepper Nuts (Pfeffernüsse)—1.4 g fat, 31.2 calories
Highest Fat: Linzertorte—23 g fat, 396.7 calories

APPLE STRUDEL *Apfelstrudel* with apples, flour, egg, oil, butter, bread crumbs, sugar, raisins, almonds, lemon rind, cinnamon, and salt

HONEY BARS *Lebkuchen* with sugar, butter, flour, almonds, candied orange, ginger, cardamom, cinnamon, and cloves

LINZERTORTE with sugar, butter, lemon rind, egg, flour, almonds, cinnamon, cloves, cocoa, and jam

MANDELTORTE with sugar, egg, orange rind, almonds, cinnamon and bread crumbs

MARZIPAN with sugar, egg white, orange juice, and almonds

PEPPER NUTS *Pfeffernüsse* with flour, molasses, butter, cinnamon, nutmeg, cloves, anise, and almonds

SACHERTORTE WITH CHOCOLATE GLAZE with semisweet chocolate, sugar, butter, bread crumbs, almonds, apricot jam, cream cheese, cream, and vanilla

Serving Size	Calories	Fat (g)	Sodium (mg)	Carbohydrate (g)	Cholesterol (mg)	Fiber (g)
6 oz	522.6	36.5	**1470.6**	10.5	163.4	0.1
6 oz	538	38	**1414.5**	10.9	176.6	0.1
6 oz	355.2	25.6	1156.8	3.3	132.4	0
6 oz	416.6	30.4	274.8	4.7	195.2	0
8 oz	601.9	42.6	511.1	6.7	193.4	0.3
1 2-inch slice	338.9	17	208.8	37.3	53.8	1.2
1 2-inch square	69.1	1.4	6.8	12.5	1.7	.06
1 3-inch wedge	396.7	**23**	176	40.7	76.7	0.7
1 2-inch wedge	122.8	9.3	44.8	5.5	137	0.3
1 oz	182	15.4	1.2	8.5	0	0.8
2 1-inch balls	31.2	1.4	18.3	3.3	5.8	0
1 2-inch slice	**405.9**	21.5	176.2	53.2	145.4	0.2

Greek and Middle Eastern Cuisine

Greek and Middle Eastern dishes are traditionally very healthy and low in fat. Both rely heavily on the use of fresh vegetables and aromatic spices. Olive oil, one of the most healthful oils available, is the predominant choice for preparing salads and sautés. Animal fats and processed foods are used very sparingly, making these cuisines a good choice for the fat-conscious diner. Meat has traditionally been a luxury in Greece and is used sparingly in Greek dishes. When it is used, it is often marinated and roasted, which makes many meat dishes lower in fat than is usually the case with other cuisines. As Greece is almost entirely surrounded by the sea, fish is an important food staple. Bean and vegetable dishes are often offered as main courses and are a good choice for people who don't want to eat too many animal products. Avoid casserole dishes prepared with butter and/or cheese, such as moussaka, spanakopita and Lebanese lamb pie, and deep-fried foods, such as fried calamari and falafel. Eat dips that contain tahini—such as baba ghanouj and hummus—in moderation since they are fairly high in fat. Follow Greek tradition and save sweets like baklava for holidays and special occasions. Greek desserts are not always high in fat but they are highly caloric since they contain lots of sugars, especially honey.

GREEK AND MIDDLE EASTERN DISHES

FOOD NAME

Appetizers and Salads
Lowest Fat: *Tzatziki—1.3 g fat, 27.3 calories*
Highest Fat: *Calamari—35.3 g fat, 477.9 calories*

BABA GHANOUJ   eggplant spread with garlic, Tahini (page 88), lemon juice, olive oil, and parsley

BEEF BOREKS   with phyllo pastry, ground beef chuck, butter, onion, garlic, tomato puree, egg yolk, parsley, cinnamon, and allspice

BEEF PATTIES WITH YOGURT SAUCE   *Keftedes*   with beef, bread, dill, cumin, egg, ouzo, fennel, and cilantro

CALAMARI   deep-fried squid with flour, salt, white pepper, and lemon juice

CHICKEN-LEMON SOUP   *Avgolemono*   with chicken broth, rice, nutmeg, and egg yolk

DOLMAS   grape leaves stuffed with ground lamb, rice, onion, and parsley

GREEK SALAD   *Horiatiki*   with tomatoes, onion, green peppers, cucumber, olive oil, oregano, feta cheese, and Greek olives

HUMMUS   Chickpea spread with Tahini (page 88), garlic, and lemon juice

PITA BREAD   with flour, salt, sugar, and vegetable shortening

SPANAKOPITA   spinach pie with onion, garlic, cilantro, oil, nutmeg, feta cheese, egg, butter, and phyllo pastry

TABBOULEH   bulgur wheat salad with celery, green pepper, tomatoes, black olives, and scallions

TARAMASALATA   fish roe with lemon juice, white bread, olive oil, and onion juice

Serving Size	Calories	Fat (g)	Sodium (mg)	Carbohydrate (g)	Cholesterol (mg)	Fiber (g)
1 tblsp	22.9	1.8	51.2	1.5	0	0.3
1 1-oz triangle	79.5	6.4	87.3	3.6	28.5	0
1 1-oz patty with two teaspoons of sauce	96.8	8	60.3	1.6	34.6	0
4 oz	**477.9**	**35.3**	326.1	15.1	276.3	0.1
1 cup	132.8	5.7	784.9	11.5	205	0
4 oz (8 small rolls)	193.9	13.6	409	16.6	49	0.5
1 ½ cups	300.5	27.4	671.7	13	12.5	2.3
1 tblsp	57.4	2.5	57.1	6.9	0	0.7
half an 8-inch bread	80	4.2	534.5	62.8	0	0.2
1 3-oz square	174	13.1	213.6	10.7	55.3	0.2
1 cup	269.4	15	356.1	21.7	18.7	0.4
1 tblsp	106.1	10.9	72.1	1.6	24	0

GREEK AND MIDDLE EASTERN DISHES

FOOD NAME

TZATZIKI cucumber and yogurt with garlic and mint

Main Dishes
Lowest Fat: Fish Plaki—13.4 g fat, 335 calories
Highest Fat: Kibbeh—70.5 g fat, 950.1 calories

AFELIA pork simmered with coriander, brown sugar and red wine

FALAFEL deep-fried chickpea croquettes with bread crumbs, paprika, parsley, marjoram, thyme, cumin, coriander, onion, garlic, egg, and Tahini

FISH PLAKI bream baked with onions, garlic, tomatoes, parsley, and oregano

LAMB-STUFFED BULGUR BALLS deep-fried with lamb shoulder, onion, parsley, salt, egg, milk, and flour

KIBBEH Lebanese lamb pie with bulgur wheat, lamb shoulder, onion, salt, cinnamon, pine nuts, currants, butter, and yogurt

KLEFTIKO Chicken baked in foil with lemon, oregano, red onions, and white wine

MOUSSAKA casserole with eggplant, ground lamb, onion, tomatoes, parsley, white wine, nutmeg, eggs, butter, flour, and milk

PASTITSIO lamb and macaroni casserole with onion, garlic, oregano, plum tomatoes, bread crumbs, Romano cheese, and cream sauce

SOFRITO veal simmered with onion, garlic, brandy, white wine, beef stock, and parsley

SOUVLAKI lamb shish kebabs with olive oil, lemon juice, garlic, oregano, green peppers, onions, mushrooms, and tomatoes

TAHINI chickpea sauce with olive oil, garlic, and spices

Serving Size	Calories	Fat (g)	Sodium (mg)	Carbohydrate (g)	Cholesterol (mg)	Fiber (g)
1 tablespoon	27.3	1.3	**906.5**	2.7	4.8	0.2
6 oz	452.4	32.1	235.6	1.2	133	0
4 2-oz balls	522.6	26.8	766	53.6	91.4	4.4
1½ cups	335	13.4	201.3	9.5	165	1
6 1-oz balls	433.8	23.8	856.8	39.6	154.9	5.9
10 oz	**950.1**	**70.5**	**1038.5**	50.1	256.8	3.2
10 oz	448.7	23.5	451	1.5	196	0.1
10 oz	754.7	60.1	403.2	11.7	238.8	0.8
12 oz	606.9	43.2	**1291.6**	18.8	170.5	0.9
5 oz	238.6	15	315.9	3.4	63.5	0.1
12 oz	**983**	65.7	526	11	196.7	1.8
1 tablespoon	51	3.78	80	2	0	0.79

GREEK AND MIDDLE EASTERN DISHES

FOOD NAME

Desserts
Lowest Fat: *Turkish Delight—1.9 g fat, 145 calories*
Highest Fat: *Halva—13.3 g fat, 309.3 calories*

BAKLAVA   phyllo pastry with honey, nuts, cinnamon, cloves, and sweet butter

HALVA   nougat with almonds, butter, sugar, and cinnamon

KADAIFI   shredded pastry with walnuts, almonds, sugar or honey, cinnamon, butter, and lemon juice

PERSIAN CREAM   with gelatin, milk, eggs, sugar, and vanilla

TURKISH DELIGHT   *Rahat Loukoum*   with fruit pectin, corn syrup, sugar, jelly, lemon rind and pistachio

Serving Size	Calories	Fat (g)	Sodium (mg)	Carbohydrate (g)	Cholesterol (mg)	Fiber (g)
1 2½-inch diamond	43.9	2.9	18.9	4	5	0.1
1 2-oz piece	309.3	13.3	0	22.7	0	0.7
1 3-inch roll	217.6	10.5	26.8	28.9	6.9	0.4
⅓ cup	332.1	12.6	174	42	303	0
1 2-inch square	145	1.9	30.9	35	0	2.1

Indian Cuisine

Since the cow is sacred in India, authentic Indian meals do not contain beef, and dairy products are scarce, with the exception of *ghee*, or clarified butter. Like other Southeast Asian cuisines, Indian menus contain lots of grains and vegetables, which in themselves have no fat. However, many Indian foods are fried, and this is not always indicated on the menu. When in doubt, ask your waitperson. Avoid coconut milk and coconut meat, both of which contain saturated fat. These are often used in a variety of dishes, including some curries. When you are in the mood for meat, an Indian restaurant is one of the best places to order it. *Tandoori* and *tikka* both indicate healthy methods of cooking. The skin and fat are removed and the meat is marinated in yoghurt and spices overnight. It is then baked in a clay oven (a *tandoor*). *Tikka* means "cube," and *tikka* on the menu indicates "boneless meat." The removal of the fat and skin from the meat not only reduces the fat content, it also removes some of the toxins that may have been in the animal's tissues, since these tend to accumulate in fat deposits. Indian cuisine also offers a variety of vegetable dishes and curries of varying spiciness. Most of these are served with rice, which provides bulk and flavor. When ordering side dishes, *nan*, a round pancake of baked bread, is a better choice than the thin, crisp *pappadums* or the fried *poori* bread often served. Nan is also wonderful for soaking up sauces during the meal. However, be sure when you order that your *nan* will not be served slathered with melted butter!

INDIAN DISHES

FOOD NAME

Breads
Lowest Fat: Chapati—4 g fat, 117 calories
Highest Fat: Parathas—19 g fat, 208 calories

CHAPATI thin bread made with white and whole-wheat flour and butter

GREEN PEA KACHORI with whole-wheat flour, cumin seeds, anise seeds, green chili, ginger and frozen peas, deep-fried in vegetable oil

NAN with white flour, egg, yogurt, butter, milk, and poppy seeds

PARATHAS multilayered bread made with white and whole-wheat flour, onion seeds, celery seeds, and butter

POORI with white and whole-wheat flour and cardamom seeds, deep-fried in vegetable oil

Appetizers and Side Dishes
Lowest Fat: Dosa—1 g fat, 77 calories
Highest Fat: Minced Lamb Patties—39 g fat, 478 calories

CHUTNEY, MANGO with red chili, cashews, raisins, mint, cumin, cayenne pepper, and coriander

CUCUMBER RAITA with cucumber, yogurt, cilantro, mint, green chili, cumin, and mustard seeds

DOSA with lentils, rice, green onions, cilantro, ginger and green chili

LIME PICKLE with fenugreek seeds, mustard seeds, chili powder, turmeric, and vegetable oil

MINCED LAMB PATTIES with lamb, lentils, onion, ground lamb, garam masala, egg, and yogurt

PRAWN KEBABS with shrimp, lime juice, vegetable oil, garlic, paprika, turmeric, green chilies and cilantro

Serving Size	Calories	Fat (g)	Sodium (mg)	Carbohydrate (g)	Cholesterol (mg)	Fiber (g)
one 5-inch bread	117	4	206	17.6	10.3	0.3
one 3-inch bread	216.1	9.9	46	29.1	0	1
one 6-inch nan	272	7	322	43.7	51.1	0.2
one 3-inch triangle	208	**19**	388	9.8	49.6	0.2
one 3-inch bread	128.3	10.4	26.9	7	0	0.1
½ cup	143.9	4.3	4.4	27.3	0	1.5
½ cup	36.7	1.7	469.7	3.6	6.4	0.2
one 4-inch cake	77	1	168	14.6	0	0.2
½ cup	92	7	**1450**	11.1	0	0.5
four 2-oz patties	**478**	**39**	80	13.4	137.8	1.1
one 3-prawn kebab	205	9	192	3.9	195	0.3

INDIAN DISHES

FOOD NAME

Rice and Vegetable Dishes
Lowest Fat: Curried Garbanzo Beans—3 g fat, 196 calories
Highest Fat: Aloo Gobi—52.3 g fat, 558 calories

ALOO GOBI   potatoes and cauliflower in curry sauce with coconut, vegetable oil, and spices

CURRIED GARBANZO BEANS   with garbanzo beans, onion, ginger, garlic, turmeric, and garam masala

DHAL BALLS WITH YOGURT   made with green lentils, yogurt, cilantro, chili powder, coconut, bread crumbs, and ginger, deep-fried in vegetable oil

FRIED RICE, FRAGRANT   with rice, cloves, cardamom, cinnamon, cumin, coriander, and onion

LENTILS, SPICED BROWN   with lentils, coconut milk, chili powder, turmeric, onion, and lemon grass

OKRA, SPICY   with okra, ginger, turmeric, chili powder, garbanzo bean flour, and yogurt

ONION BHAJJIS   with garbanzo bean flour, coriander, cumin, green chilies, onions, and cilantro, deep-fried in vegetable oil

RICE, SWEET SAFFRON   with rice, cloves, cardamom, cinnamon, raisins, and sugar

Curry Dishes
Lowest Fat: Mushroom Curry—6 g fat, 87 calories
Highest Fat: Hot-and-Sour Pork Curry—59 g fat, 679 calories

CURRY, CHICKEN AND APRICOT   with chicken, garam masala, ginger, garlic, onions, apricots, and tomatoes

CURRY, DRY POTATO   with potatoes, mustard seeds, onion, garlic, ginger, green chilies, turmeric, and cumin

Serving Size	Calories	Fat (g)	Sodium (mg)	Carbohydrate (g)	Cholesterol (mg)	Fiber (g)
1¼ cups	**558**	**52.3**	294.1	36.5	0	8.2
½ cup	196	3	515	32.6	0	2.6
six 1-inch balls	270	15	**952**	30.7	75.8	1.2
1 cup	326	11	507	52.3	0	0.4
¾ cup	154	7	21	18.2	0	0.9
1 cup	143	9	542	11.2	9.1	1
4 small balls (½ cup)	143	10	503	9.9	0	0.9
1 cup	457	11	511	70.9	0	0.4
1 cup	444	23.5	368	27.8	115.8	1.4
half-cup	133	7	506	16.4	0	0.7

INDIAN DISHES

FOOD NAME

CURRY, FISH WITH SAFFRON with white fish fillets, saffron, garlic, ginger, turmeric, coriander, garam masala, garbanzo bean flour, yogurt and whipping cream

CURRY, HOT-AND-SOUR PORK with boneless pork shoulder (simmered), hot spice mix, vinegar, brown sugar, ginger, and garlic

CURRY, KASHMIR MEATBALL with ground lamb, garam masala, cayenne pepper, yogurt, cinnamon, cardamom, and ginger

CURRY, MADRAS MEAT with beef round steak, onion, cloves, chilies, ginger, and cardamom

CURRY, MIXED VEGETABLE with onion, cumin, chili powder, potatoes, cauliflower, green beans, carrots, and tomatoes

CURRY, MUSHROOM with mushrooms, green chilies, coriander, cumin, garlic, coconut milk, and butter

CURRY, RED LAMB AND ALMOND with boneless lamb, onion, almonds, cardamom, turmeric, chili powder, nut masala, yogurt and tomatoes

CURRY, SHRIMP AND FISH BALL with white fish, bread crumbs, eggs, cilantro, lemon juice, onion, green chilies, garlic, coconut milk, and tomatoes, deep-fried in vegetable oil

Beef, Lamb and Pork Dishes
Lowest Fat: *Lamb Tikka—32 g fat, 440 calories*
Highest Fat: *Beef Kebabs—51 g fat, 627 calories*

BEEF KEBABS with beef, onion, ginger, garlic, chili powder, garam masala, cilantro, almonds, eggs, and yogurt

LAMB KORMA with lamb, onion, nut masala, garam masala, red chilies, ginger, and half-and-half

LAMB TIKKA with lamb, cumin, turmeric, yogurt, onion, ginger, garlic, and garam masala

Serving Size	Calories	Fat (g)	Sodium (mg)	Carbohydrate (g)	Cholesterol (mg)	Fiber (g)
1½ cups	357	20	673	8.5	109.6	0.4
1 cup	**679**	**59**	111	7.7	123.4	0.3
four 2-ounce meatballs	496	42	588	2.5	104	0.1
1⅛ cups	423	28	534	6.9	89.3	0.9
1½ cups	183	11	174	20.7	0	1.6
one cup	87	6	572	7.5	15.5	0.7
1½ cups	**792**	38	115	8.9	104.2	0.6
six 2-ounce balls	389	20	**1298**	26	235	1
one kebab with four 2½-ounce cubes	**627**	**51**	145	5.9	215.2	0.4
1¼ cups	538	44	617	7.7	121.6	0.6
8 ounces	440	32	713	1.8	135.2	.04

INDIAN DISHES

FOOD NAME

LAMB WITH CAULIFLOWER   with lamb, cauliflower, onions, ginger, garlic, hot spice mix, beef stock, and garam masala
LAMB VINDALOO   with lamb, chilies, peppercorns, cumin, ginger, garlic, vinegar, tamarind pulp, anise, and cloves
LAMB WITH ONIONS   with lamb, onions, turmeric, cumin, coriander, onions, potatoes, and garam masala
SPARE RIBS   spare ribs with hot spices, turmeric, ginger, onion, and tomato paste

Chicken Dishes
Lowest Fat: *Chicken with Lentils—20 g fat, 307 calories*
Highest Fat: *Lemon and Coriander Chicken—46 g fat, 609 calories*

CHICKEN BIRIYANI   with chicken, cardamom, cumin, onions, garlic, ginger, yogurt, rice, saffron, and almonds
CHICKEN IN GINGER SAUCE   chicken with garlic, cumin, garam masala, and lemon juice
CHICKEN TIKKA   with chicken, yogurt, ginger, garlic, chili powder, coriander, and lime juice
CHICKEN VINDALOO   with chicken, chilies, peppercorns, cumin, ginger, garlic, vinegar, tamarind pulp, anise, and cloves
CHICKEN WITH LENTILS   with chicken, lentils, turmeric, cardamom, onion, ginger, cumin, and garlic
LEMON AND CORIANDER CHICKEN   with chicken, lemon, coriander, ginger, garlic, green chili, turmeric, cumin, and cayenne pepper
TANDOORI CHICKEN   with chicken, lime juice, onion, tandoori masala, garam masala, ginger, and yogurt

Serving Size	Calories	Fat (g)	Sodium (mg)	Carbohydrate (g)	Cholesterol (mg)	Fiber (g)
1¼ cups	536	45	830	7.9	101.3	0.6
1¼ cups	487.5	40.3	358	3.7	99.4	0.3
1½ cups	672	45	587	39.7	101.3	1.4
6 ribs (10 oz)	513	42	135	2.5	136.3	0.1
1 cup	541.5	21	312	63.3	51.2	0.4
1 cup	396	26	617	2.7	117	0.3
3 short skewers (8 oz)	411	27	632	3	121.8	.04
1 cup	497.7	34.2	407.1	4.7	147	0.3
1 cup	307	20	541	15.3	39	0.4
1 thigh and 1 drumstick	**609**	**46**	697	2.7	203.4	.29
10 oz	490.9	29.7	264.2	4.9	193.1	.08

INDIAN DISHES

FOOD NAME

Seafood Dishes
Lowest Fat: Fish Kebabs with Coriander—3 g fat, 192 calories
Highest Fat: Fish in Hot Sauce—45 g fat, 606 calories

COD STEAKS, SPICED WITH COCONUT with cod, onion, coconut, ginger, garlic, green chilies, lemon, cilantro, and tomato

FISH IN HOT SAUCE with whole mackerel, dill, lime, green onions, ginger, garlic, mustard seeds, tamarind paste, and tomato paste

FISH KEBABS WITH CORIANDER with monkfish fillet, yogurt, garlic, garam masala, coriander, green chilies, green onions, and lime

FISH, STEAMED WITH VEGETABLES with whole red snapper, garam masala, turmeric, cilantro, parsley, ginger, new potatoes, carrots, and zucchini

FISH WITH CILANTRO AND CHILE with monkfish, lemon juice, cilantro, green chilies, garlic, and yogurt, deep-fried in vegetable oil

HOT MUSSELS WITH CUMIN with mussels, cumin, onion, ginger, garlic, green chilies, turmeric, coconut, and cilantro

MADRAS CURRIED CRAB with crab, onion, garlic, ginger, tomato, green chilies, coconut, nut masala, and coconut milk

SHRIMP AND MUSTARD SEEDS with shrimp, mustard seeds, turmeric, cayenne pepper, green chilies, and butter

SHRIMP PATTIES, SPICY with shrimp, white fish fillets, green onions, ginger, cilantro, mint, bread crumbs, egg, lemon juice, garbanzo bean flour, and coriander

SOLE, SPICED AND GRILLED Sole with yogurt, garlic, garam masala, coriander, chili powder, and lemon juice

SOLE WITH DILL STUFFING Sole with lemon juice, garlic, cayenne pepper, turmeric, dill, and green onions

Serving Size	Calories	Fat (g)	Sodium (mg)	Carbohydrate (g)	Cholesterol (mg)	Fiber (g)
9 oz	199	18	609	10.1	74	1.6
one 8-oz fish	**606**	**45**	209	5.5	160	0.4
7 oz	192	3	658	5.1	86.8	0.3
one 8-oz fish	352	10	660	15.1	82.6	0.7
9 oz	294	11	694	6.8	102.9	0.6
15 mussels (12 oz)	259	21	91	12.6	38.3	1.8
1 medium crab	304	14	**1444**	10.2	70	0.9
4 oz	173	8	727	1.7	188.8	0.1
four 2-inch round patties	420	26	**1447**	24.7	174	0.7
one 8-oz fillet	234	4	703	2.5	114.1	0.1
one 8-oz fillet	213	7	642	2.8	82	0.4

INDIAN DISHES

FOOD NAME

Desserts
Lowest Fat: Pistachio Halva—5 g fat, 74 calories
Highest Fat: Coconut Pancakes—25 g fat, 413 calories

CARDAMOM AND NUT ICE CREAM with whole milk, cardamom pods, almonds, and pistachios

COCONUT PANCAKES with coconut, flour, brown sugar, fresh coconut, ginger root, anise and yogurt

FRITTERS AND FRAGRANT SYRUP with flour, cardamom, rose water, saffron, yogurt, butter, and raisins, deep-fried in vegetable oil

PISTACHIO HALVA with pistachios, whole milk, butter, and vanilla

SAFFRON RICE PUDDING with basmati rice, whole milk, butter, cardamom pods, cinnamon, cloves, raisins, and almonds

Serving Size	Calories	Fat (g)	Sodium (mg)	Carbohydrate (g)	Cholesterol (mg)	Fiber (g)
4 oz	328	19	161	28.9	44	0.3
two 7-inch pancakes	**413**	**25**	322	40.3	78.8	2.1
two 1-inch balls	405.9	15.8	146.1	53.6	10.3	0.3
one 2-inch square	74	5	10	6.8	2.5	0.2
1 cup	461	13	78	65.8	18.2	0.6

Italian Cuisine

Italian cooking makes great use of olive oil, garlic, and onions, all of which are considered extremely healthy—olive oil because of its blood cholesterol-lowering properties, garlic for its various medicinal qualities, and onions for their nutrients and fiber. The other Italian mainstay, of course, is pasta. As a grain product, pasta is generally a healthful staple, providing complex carbohydrates and important nutrients with a minimum of fat. However, all pasta products are not created equal; egg noodles have a higher fat content than plain wheat pasta, and any pasta dish can become quite fatty when buried in creamy sauces or sausage toppings. Any dish called "Parmigiana" is made with liberal amounts of Parmesan cheese and is not a good low-fat choice; dishes called "marsala" or "piccata" are usually lower in fat. Choose fresh tomatoes on angel hair pasta, or spaghetti marinara without meatballs. In general, choose red pasta sauces rather than white. Indulge in green, not Caesar, salad (which is made with eggs), or try a plate of fresh, not deep-fried, vegetables as a side dish. Fresh Italian bread or bread sticks are delicious, and good choices without butter; garlic bread often is made with a fatty spread. Since Italy is surrounded by water on three sides, Italian cooks are no strangers to seafood, and fish and shellfish can be particularly satisfying as an alternative to meat. Note the cooking method, however; choose poaching, broiling, or steaming over frying or sautéing.

ITALIAN DISHES

FOOD NAME

Appetizers

Lowest Fat: Onions Baked in Balsamic Vinegar—0.1 g fat, 13 calories

Highest Fat: Rice Croquettes with Sausage—102.3 g fat-1217.6 calories

---

ANCHOVY DIP WITH VEGETABLES *Bagna Cauda* with butter, olive oil, anchovies, and garlic

ANTIPASTO ALLA RUSTICA Provolone cheese and salami salad with vinaigrette

BAKED FONTINA CHEESE WITH MARINATED ARTICHOKES with cheese, artichokes, butter and olive oil

BAKED SMOKED MOZZARELLA WITH PICKLED MUSHROOMS with mozzarella, pickled mushrooms, and served with crusty bread

BEANS COOKED IN THE STYLE OF LITTLE BIRDS *Fagioli agli Uccelli* with beans, black-eyed peas, sage, and tomatoes

CAPONATA fried eggplant with tomatoes, olives, and capers

CAPONATA WITH RED AND GREEN PEPPERS as above, with peppers

CAULIFLOWER FRITTI cauliflower fried in bread crumbs and served with marinara sauce

CHICKEN LIVER PÂTÉ WITH MARSALA with chicken livers, marsala, and served on crostini

CHICKEN LIVER PÂTÉ WITH PISTACHIOS ROLLED IN PROSCIUTTO with chicken livers, pistachios, olive oil, and prosciutto; served on crostini

CHICKPEA FRITTERS with chickpea flour, salt, and parsley

CHICKPEAS WITH MUSTARD-SAGE DRESSING with chick peas, mayonnaise, Dijon mustard, parsley, and sage

Serving Size	Calories	Fat (g)	Sodium (mg)	Carbohydrate (g)	Cholesterol (mg)	Fiber (g)
3 oz vegetables and 2½ tblsp dip	431.2	44.7	253.5	7.3	20.7	104
7 oz	283.9	25.9	810.8	2	32	.06
3 oz	411.6	22.1	319.3	33.5	73.8	0.2
3 oz	303.5	16.4	473.5	23.8	51.8	.25
8 oz	194.8	7.8	277.3	24	0	0.5
¾ cup	86.8	6.3	391.5	7.9	0	1.1
¾ cup	46.5	3.8	823.7	3.6	0	0.5
1½ cups	719	60.6	**1182.3**	34.8	109.6	2
4 oz	472.9	30.8	716.4	24.6	399.4	.09
4 oz	441.4	27.9	778	27.2	255.8	0.2
7 oz	586.3	50.4	248.4	27.1	0	2.2
3 oz	323.1	15.6	160.2	35.6	0	2.9

ITALIAN DISHES

FOOD NAME

CHICKPEAS WITH RED ONIONS AND PESTO   with chickpeas, red onions, garlic, basil, oil, pine nuts, and lemon
CROSTINI   appetizer toast with olive oil
CROSTINI CAPONATA   appetizer toast with eggplant spread
CROSTINI WITH BEL PAESE CHEESE AND ANCHOVIES   with olive oil and butter
FONTINA AND VERMOUTH DIP   with butter and dry vermouth
FRIED EGGPLANT AND ZUCCHINI STICKS   with eggplant, zucchini, flour, eggs, bread crumbs, salt, and cayenne pepper
FRIED PROVOLONE   with provolone cheese, flour, eggs, and bread crumbs
FRIED TORTELLINI   tortellini served with pesto
GARLIC SPREAD, ROASTED   garlic, olive oil
ITALIAN CHEESE FONDUE   *Fondutta*   with Fontina cheese, butter, milk, egg yolks, nutmeg, and bread cubes
KIDNEY BEANS WITH SALAMI AND SCALLIONS   with kidney beans, salami, scallions, olive oil and vinegar
KIDNEY BEANS WITH SHRIMP   with kidney beans, shrimp, oregano, lemon, hot pepper, and vinaigrette
MARINATED CARROTS   carrots with salami in vinaigrette
MARINATED EGGPLANT SALAD   with eggplant, olive oil, basil, and mint
MARINATED MUSHROOMS   mushrooms with lemon, oregano, vinegar, olive oil, and onion
MOZZARELLA MARINATED WITH BASIL AND SUN-DRIED TOMATOES   mozzarella with basil, sun-dried tomatoes, and olive oil

Serving Size	Calories	Fat (g)	Sodium (mg)	Carbohydrate (g)	Cholesterol (mg)	Fiber (g)
4 oz	373.2	16.1	98.8	43.2	4.8	3.5
2 oz	130.2	6.9	154.7	14.8	0	0
3 oz	176.3	10.2	477.9	18.9	0	.5
3 oz	381.1	27.2	456.8	22.6	53.7	0
3 oz	421.8	27.8	133.8	20.1	89.3	.05
9 oz	**1004.5**	**93.1**	381.8	30.3	102.8	1
7 oz	**1025**	**90.5**	937.3	18.3	146.9	.09
4 oz	612.7	63.3	142.4	8.4	8.5	.09
2 tablespoons	31.9	1.9	4	3.6	0	0.2
8 oz	459.6	34.2	227.8	15.5	318.7	0
3 oz	146.8	8.2	153.4	13.7	2.7	1
⅔ cup	197.8	8.1	271.7	15.1	86.7	1.1
3½ oz	98.3	8.9	175.2	3.4	4	0.4
⅔ cup	145.5	14.8	583.1	3.6	0	0.6
⅔ cup	118.5	12.2	239.6	2.7	0	0.9
2 oz	203.1	19	112.7	2.3	22	0.7

ITALIAN DISHES

FOOD NAME
MOZZARELLA MARINATED WITH CAPERS AND ANCHOVIES mozzarella, capers, and anchovies served with fresh parsley and tomatoes
MOZZARELLA ROLLED WITH GORGONZOLA AND BASIL with mozzarella, gorgonzola and basil
MUSHROOM AND SHRIMP ANTIPASTO with mushrooms, shrimp, mayonnaise, basil, and tomato
MUSHROOM SALAD with mushrooms, lemon juice, olive oil, garlic, and oregano
ONIONS BAKED IN BALSAMIC VINEGAR onions with sugar and balsamic vinegar
OLIVES MARINATED WITH CAPERS with olives, capers, olive oil, and spices
OLIVES, SPICY MARINATED olives in hot pepper and garlic vinaigrette
PARMESAN PUFFS with Italian bread, parmesan cheese, olive oil, mayonnaise, and Worcestershire sauce
PIEDMONTESE SPREAD WITH MASCARPONE, GORGONZOLA, AND WALNUTS served with crostini
RED BELL PEPPERS red peppers roasted with garlic and olive oil
RICE CROQUETTES WITH PARMESAN AND MOZZARELLA CHEESE with butter, onions, chicken stock, eggs, bread crumbs, and tomato sauce
RICE CROQUETTES WITH SAUSAGE *Arancini* with chicken stock, Parmesan, mozzarella, butter, eggs, olive oil, tomato paste, and bread crumbs
SICILIAN CAPONATA fried eggplant with pine nuts and raisins
STUFFED MUSHROOMS with mushrooms, bread crumbs, Parmesan cheese, butter, olive oil, onions, garlic, prosciutto, and marjoram

Serving Size	Calories	Fat (g)	Sodium (mg)	Carbohydrate (g)	Cholesterol (mg)	Fiber (g)
2 oz	199.1	18.5	255.3	2	22	0.1
6 oz	331.6	29.5	521.3	2.6	93.4	0
4 oz	176.9	13.6	171.8	3.4	74.3	0.6
4 oz	80.2	8.2	215.4	1.7	0	0.8
3 oz	13	0.1	0.5	3.9	0	0.1
2 oz	70.4	7.8	84	0.6	0	0.3
4 oz	123.8	13.2	192.7	2.4	0	0.7
3 oz (two slices)	350.7	28.8	543.1	16.1	9.5	0
½ cup	446	36.2	461.3	22.1	70.4	0.2
6 oz	72.8	7	91.2	3	0	0.6
12 oz	**1094.6**	**87.7**	**2207.9**	51.7	134.1	1.7
12 oz	**1217.6**	**102.3**	**1987.1**	43.2	177.7	0.2
5 oz	175.3	12.2	851.2	12.7	0	1
2 large mushrooms	132.1	9	664.2	5.1	22.8	0.7

ITALIAN DISHES

FOOD NAME

STUFFED MUSSELS   mussels with bread crumbs, parsley, onion, olive oil, and hot pepper flakes

SWEET PEPPERS WITH ROSEMARY, GARLIC, AND RICOTTA SALATA   with red, yellow, and green bell peppers, rosemary, garlic, ricotta, and olive oil

SAUTEED BROCCOLI RABE   with broccoli, garlic, olive oil and salt

TUSCAN WHITE BEAN SALAD   with rosemary, sage, celery, onions, and olive oil

RED OR YELLOW PEPPERS WITH BASIL, ROASTED   peppers with basil, olive oil, and garlic

Breads, Pizzas and Sandwiches
Lowest Fat: Bread Sticks—10 g fat, 178 calories
Highest Fat: Sausage and Cheese Calzone—35 g fat, 734.5 calories

BREAD STICKS   with sesame and poppy seeds and hot pepper flakes

CALZONE, SAUSAGE AND CHEESE   with sausage, marinara sauce, fennel seeds, mozzarella, and Parmesan cheese

FOCACCIA WITH ROSEMARY AND GARLIC   with olive oil, garlic, parmesan cheese, and rosemary

GARLIC BREAD   Italian bread topped with butter and garlic

HERO SANDWICH, MEATBALL   meatballs on Italian bread with Romano and mozzarella cheeses

HERO SANDWICH WITH SAUSAGE AND PEPPERS   with sausage, fennel sausage, onions, bell peppers, and tomatoes on Italian rolls

PANINI, PROSCIUTTO AND CHEESE   thin sandwiches grilled in butter, with Fontina cheese and prosciutto

PIZZA MARGHERITA   with marinara sauce, mozzarella, Parmesan, and basil

Serving Size	Calories	Fat (g)	Sodium (mg)	Carbohydrate (g)	Cholesterol (mg)	Fiber (g)
4 medium mussels	237	8.6	410	13.1	54.9	.04
6 oz	119.6	11.5	14.9	2.9	7.8	0.5
4 oz	89.5	7.2	211.8	5.3	0	.63
½-cup	53.4	3.1	716.2	5	0	0.4
6 oz	61.3	6	77.9	2.3	0	0.5
1¼ oz	178	10	933	18.9	0	0.4
9 oz	**734.5**	**35**	**1911.5**	69.5	89	1.01
3 oz	284	10	382	28.6	0	0.3
3 oz	234	14	368	23.4	33.8	.03
9 oz	409	22	847	33.9	90.6	0.3
12 oz	432	22	**1150**	39.3	52	0.7
3 oz	332	27	724.4	24.3	63.7	0
1 5-oz slice	411.4	19.8	869.3	30.2	24.2	0.1

ITALIAN DISHES

FOOD NAME

PIZZA, PEPPERONCINI AND PEPPERONI with marinara sauce, garlic, pepperoni, pepperoncini, and mozzarella and Parmesan cheeses

PIZZA, WHITE *Pizza Bianco* with basil, garlic, and mozzarella, Fontina, and Parmesan cheeses

PIZZA WITH ARTICHOKES AND SUN-DRIED TOMATOES topped with artichokes, sun-dried tomatoes, oregano, garlic, and mozzarella and Parmesan cheeses

Soups
Lowest Fat: Spinach Soup—1.3 g fat, 47.3 calories
Highest Fat: Lentil Soup—16 g fat, 218.6 calories

CHICKPEA-ESCAROLE SOUP with chickpeas, escarole, tomatoes, chicken stock, and salt pork

FIVE-BEAN SOUP with white beans, kidney beans, cranberry beans, lentils, and green split peas with salt pork, tomatoes, and cabbage

CLAM SOUP with whole fresh clams, white wine, and clam juice

GARLIC SOUP with garlic, bread cubes, red wine, chicken stock, and eggs

LENTIL SOUP with lentils, onions, carrots, ham hock, and oregano

LENTIL SOUP WITH PASTA with lentils, pasta and chicken stock

MACARONI AND BEAN with chicken stock, macaroni, white beans, and tomatoes

MEATBALL SOUP with ground chuck, beef broth, and pastina

MINESTRONE GENOA STYLE with white beans, tomatoes, ham hock, cabbage, zucchini, and pesto

MINESTRONE, NEAPOLITAN with Italian sausage, salt pork, chicken stock, carrots, tomatoes, cabbage, and macaroni

Serving Size	Calories	Fat (g)	Sodium (mg)	Carbohydrate (g)	Cholesterol (mg)	Fiber (g)
1 5-oz slice	494	26.7	1298	29.3	44.2	0.9
1 5-oz slice	444.5	23.6	476.8	24.6	46.2	0.2
1 5-oz slice	414.5	19.4	839	30.6	24.2	1
1 cup	227.4	7.3	753	27.1	12.7	2.2
1 cup	107.2	3.3	322.1	13.3	7.9	0.9
1 cup	252.1	9.3	360.9	18.9	44.5	.03
1 cup	216.3	12	934.7	12	230.8	.08
1 cup	218.6	**16**	74.6	5.8	41.6	0.4
1 cup	145.1	6.2	968.7	12.4	3.6	0.5
1 cup	113.6	4.9	91.8	10.3	2.7	0.5
1 cup	121.5	8.2	**858.2**	3.2	23.6	.01
1 cup	239.9	15	98	15.5	31.1	1.3
1 cup	241.2	15.6	**1194.9**	9.1	39.4	0.5

ITALIAN DISHES

FOOD NAME

MINESTRONE WITH DRY AND FRESH BEANS   with salt pork, cranberry beans, green beans, tomatoes, and carrots

PASTINA AND EGG SOUP   with chicken stock, nutmeg, and Parmesan cheese

SPINACH SOUP   with chicken stock

TOMATO AND BREAD SOUP   with chicken stock, garlic, and basil

TOMATO SOUP   with chicken stock, onions, and rice

TUSCAN BEAN SOUP   with white beans, ham hock, and Parmesan cheese

VEGETABLE SOUP   *Aguacotta*   with tomatoes, onions, peppers, eggs, Parmesan cheese, and croutons

Salads
Lowest Fat: *Spinach Salad—11.4 g fat, 190 calories*
Highest Fat: *Caesar Salad—31.8 g fat, 354.4 calories*

CAESAR SALAD   with romaine lettuce, croutons, anchovies, and Parmesan cheese

COLD CALAMARI SALAD   with squid, red onion, celery, tomatoes, garlic, lime juice, salt, pepper, olive oil, and parsley

SPINACH SALAD   with spinach, mushrooms, scallions, bacon, egg, vinegar, and sugar

Beef and Pork Dishes
Lowest Fat: *Meat Balls in Mushroom Sauce—18.9 g fat, 285 calories*
Highest Fat: *Pork and Sausages Contadina—55.9 g fat, 1138.7 calories*

MEAT BALLS IN MUSHROOM SAUCE   with lean ground beef, bread crumbs, eggs, nutmeg, onions, garlic, tomatoes, peppers, celery, and mushrooms

Serving Size	Calories	Fat (g)	Sodium (mg)	Carbohydrate (g)	Cholesterol (mg)	Fiber (g)
1 cup	95.9	4.5	530.7	9.1	10.7	0.8
1 cup	144.1	8.5	700.1	6.3	144.8	.02
1½ cups	47.3	1.3	808.7	4	.07	0.2
1 cup	94.2	2.7	622.4	12.9	0.6	0.6
1 cup	65.9	1.3	703.7	8.7	0.7	0.6
1½ cups	188.4	10.1	181.4	15	26.2	0.7
1 cup	142.6	7.9	520.7	13.3	93.5	0.6
1½ cups	**354.4**	**31.8**	**1223.3**	10.5	74.4	0.6
¾ cup	375.1	21.6	872.8	17.1	386.8	.57
1½ cups	78.3	4.1	152.5	6	72.5	1
8 oz	285	18.9	705	12.9	92	2.7

ITALIAN DISHES

FOOD NAME

MIXED BOIL *Bollito Misto* with beef brisket, lamb tongues, Italian sausage, chicken, turnips, cabbage and potatoes

PORK SAUSAGES CONTADINA with pork sausages, onion, zucchini, peppers, carrots, and vinegar, and served with polenta

PORK, ROASTED, WITH FENNEL Pork with olive oil, fennel, and onions

Chicken and Poultry Dishes
Lowest Fat: Quail Flambéed with Brandy—19.1 g fat, 565.2 calories
Highest Fat: Roast Duck with Fresh Cherries and Chianti—117.2 g fat, 1253.5 calories

CHICKEN BREASTS WITH ARTICHOKES, CREAM AND TOMATOES chicken breasts with artichoke hearts, onion, white wine, chicken broth, cream, tomatoes, and basil

CHICKEN BREASTS WITH WALNUTS AND GORGONZOLA with chicken breasts, walnuts, gorgonzola cheese, chicken stock, heavy cream, and basil

CHICKEN CACCIATORA chicken with olive oil, onions, garlic, red wine, tomatoes, oregano, and parsley

CHICKEN MARSALA chicken with butter, olive oil, onion, Marsala wine, and chicken stock

CHICKEN ROLLATINI WITH PESTO chicken with prosciutto and mozzarella

CHICKEN SALTIMBOCCA chicken with prosciutto, sage, and white wine

CHICKEN SCALOPPINE WITH LEMON AND CAPERS chicken with white wine and chicken stock

Serving Size	Calories	Fat (g)	Sodium (mg)	Carbohydrate (g)	Cholesterol (mg)	Fiber (g)
16 oz	663.7	42.9	**1567.5**	18.9	169.8	1.5
14 oz	**1138.7**	**55.9**	**1066.1**	98.9	184	3.2
11 oz	722.7	52.8	456.9	2.6	202.7	0.3
13 oz	753.9	35.3	890.7	12.4	293.6	0.6
12 oz	977.9	48.4	940.5	3.8	381.3	0.4
10 oz (2 pieces of chicken)	486.2	30.4	597.4	6.6	165.6	0.5
10 oz (2 pieces of chicken)	651.1	44.7	**1224.4**	9.2	205	.07
8 oz	604.8	33.1	587.2	12.2	233.6	.09
12 oz (2 breast pieces)	690.1	**27.2**	**1004.4**	2.6	303.4	0
10 oz (2 breast pieces)	465.2	19.3	667.1	2.6	183.1	0

ITALIAN DISHES

FOOD NAME

CHICKEN WITH GREEN OLIVES chicken with red wine, tomatoes, and olives

CHICKEN ROASTED WITH LEMON AND ROSEMARY chicken breasts rubbed with olive oil, lemon, and rosemary

CHICKEN STUFFED WITH SAUSAGE AND MOZZARELLA

CORNISH GAME HEN STUFFED WITH DRIED FIGS AND PEARS Cornish hen with olive oil and port wine

DUCK, ROAST, WITH FRESH CHERRIES AND CHIANTI duck with onion, garlic, and celery

QUAIL FLAMBÉED WITH BRANDY quail with French bread, butter, olive oil, and garlic

TURKEY SCALOPPINE WITH PANCETTA AND MOZZARELLA CHEESE Turkey with pancetta, mozzarella, olive oil and tomato sauce

Pasta, Polenta and Rice Dishes
Lowest Fat: Fettuccine in Sun-Cooked Tomato Sauce—4.6 g fat, 296.2 calories
Highest Fat: Ricotta-Stuffed Ravioli with Walnut Sauce—75.9 g fat, 1207.4 calories

ANGEL HAIR PASTA AND LEMON PARSLEY SAUCE Pasta with garlic, olive oil, and Parmesan cheese

ANGEL HAIR PASTA WITH SCALLOPS MARINARA Pasta with white wine, tomatoes and basil

CANNELLONI STUFFED WITH CHICKEN, HAM, AND MUSHROOMS Pasta with chicken, ham, and mushrooms, topped with Béchamel Sauce

EGGPLANT PARMESAN with eggplant, bread crumbs, mushrooms, mozzarella, parmesan, eggs, paprika, and tomato sauce

Serving Size	Calories	Fat (g)	Sodium (mg)	Carbohydrate (g)	Cholesterol (mg)	Fiber (g)
14 oz	830.6	43.9	768.7	6.7	326.7	0.8
10 oz	858.3	47	**1012.3**	0.9	367.5	.04
12 oz	937	52.3	717.3	9.2	364.4	.03
1 12-oz hen	822.5	23.7	576.2	37.3	298.6	2.8
14 oz	**1253.5**	**117.2**	723.8	14.8	218	0.5
8 oz	565.2	19.1	363.9	6.5	5.9	.01
7 oz	564.6	42.3	1000.2	9.1	124.3	1.3
1 cup	582.6	16.7	882.7	81.1	14.3	0.2
1½ cups	474.8	6.7	440.2	69.6	22.4	0.4
14 oz	796	34.1	**1654.6**	62.5	161.5	0.4
12 oz	500.8	31.9	1767	33.1	149.8	2.8

ITALIAN DISHES

FOOD NAME

FETTUCCINE ALFREDO fettuccine pasta with butter, heavy cream, and Parmesan cheese

FETTUCCINE IN SUN-COOKED TOMATO SAUCE fettuccine pasta with tomato, onion, basil, and parsley marinated in olive oil

FETTUCCINE WITH CREAM, PROSCIUTTO, AND PEAS fettuccine pasta with butter, cream, prosciutto, peas, and Parmesan cheese

FETTUCCINE WITH MUSHROOMS AND SHRIMP fettuccine pasta with fresh and dried mushrooms, shrimp, white wine, heavy cream, and butter

FETTUCCINE WITH PESTO fettuccine pasta with basil, garlic, walnuts, Parmesan cheese, and butter

FETTUCCINE WITH SPINACH AND CREAM fettuccine pasta with spinach, butter, basil, and Parmesan cheese

FUSILLI WITH ARTICHOKES fusilli pasta with artichokes, garlic, tomatoes, basil, and Romano cheese

FUSILLI WITH FRESH TOMATOES AND CHEESE fusilli pasta with ricotta salata or feta cheese

FUSILLI WITH LAMB AND TOMATO RAGÙ fusilli pasta with lamb, red wine, garlic, rosemary, and parsley

FUSILLI WITH TUNA fusilli pasta with tomatoes, capers, and canned tuna in oil

GNOCCHI ALLA ROMANA with semolina flour, Parmesan cheese, milk, and egg yolks

GNOCCHI, POTATO with potato, egg yolks and flour

LASAGNE with lasagne pasta, beef chuck, tomatoes, Italian sausage, and ricotta, Parmesan, and mozzarella cheeses

LINGUINE WITH GARLIC PESTO linguine pasta with garlic, basil, pine nuts, Romano cheese, Parmesan cheese, and olive oil

Serving Size	Calories	Fat (g)	Sodium (mg)	Carbohydrate (g)	Cholesterol (mg)	Fiber (g)
1 cup	644.9	37.6	513.5	47.3	136	0
1¼ cups	296.2	4.6	88.1	52	0	0.7
1 cup	586.8	32.8	665.5	50.3	112.3	0.5
10 oz	384.3	11	265.7	46.7	106.4	0.3
1 cup	601.4	36.1	716.6	47.1	36.3	0.2
1 cup	532.4	29	674.9	47.5	95	.07
1¼ cups	387.3	6.8	246.3	66.2	4.8	1
1¼ cups	359.5	13.9	296.1	45.6	11.6	0.6
1½ cups	370.9	19.3	314.6	29	45	0.5
1½ cups	349.4	7.3	116.6	50.5	18.6	0.7
1¼ cups	463.4	36	**1465**	15.2	207.6	0.7
1¼ cups	341.7	3	365.3	54.6	90.7	1
16 oz	822.4	51	**1208.5**	409	257.9	0.9
1 cup	687	45.7	328	48.5	22	0.3

ITALIAN DISHES

FOOD NAME

LINGUINE WITH RED CLAM SAUCE   linguine pasta with clams in shells, olive oil, garlic, tomatoes, parsley, and oregano
LINGUINE WITH WHITE CLAM SAUCE
ORECCHIETTE WITH SWISS CHARD   orecchiette pasta with anchovies, garlic, hot pepper, and Romano and Parmesan cheeses
PASTA PRIMAVERA   linguine pasta with asparagus, carrots, and peas
PASTA PUTTANESCA   with linguine, olive oil, anchovy, garlic, tomatoes, capers, black olives, oregano and salt
PASTA WITH CREAM, WALNUTS, AND GORGONZOLA CHEESE
PENNE WITH PORK AND TOMATO SAUCE   penne pasta with olive oil, onions, carrots, celery, garlic, tomatoes, Romano and Parmesan cheese
PENNE WITH SQUID   penne pasta with squid, pancetta, red wine, and tomatoes
PENNE WITH TUNA   penne pasta with pimientos, olives, canned tuna, and vinaigrette
POLENTA   with cornmeal, salt, butter, and Parmesan cheese
POLENTA BROILED WITH SAGE AND ROSEMARY   polenta with Parmesan cheese, sage, and rosemary
POLENTA WITH SAGE AND FONTINA   polenta with butter and Parmesan cheese, sage, and Fontina cheese
POLENTA WITH SAUSAGE RAGÙ   with sausage, butter, Parmesan and mozzarella cheeses
RAVIOLI WITH BASIL AND HAZELNUTS   pasta with butter, basil, and hazelnuts

Serving Size	Calories	Fat (g)	Sodium (mg)	Carbohydrate (g)	Cholesterol (mg)	Fiber (g)
10 oz pasta, 12 clams	708	8.5	554.5	95.6	80	1.1
1¼ cups pasta, 12 clams	589	12.4	158.1	69.4	76.4	.03
1¼ cups	499.2	18.8	**1001.3**	54.1	42.3	0.1
1½ cups	329.7	7.2	647.1	50.7	16.3	0.9
1½ cups	320.1	11.7	245.6	43.4	0.0	.61
¾ cup	536.1	31	357.8	47.7	87.9	0.2
1½ cups	704.4	35.6	764.2	56.2	97.9	1.01
1½ cups	681.8	18.3	**1066.4**	78.9	365	0.6
1¼ cups	553.9	21.8	661.3	63.8	20.8	0.5
10 oz	330.2	19.8	367.5	33.9	26.5	0.6
10 oz	228.7	10.3	919	25.7	24.1	0.3
11 oz	351.9	21.1	952.4	26	61.3	0.3
13 oz	477.4	27.9	**1853.7**	34.3	72	1.4
¾ cup	535.8	31	166.4	50.1	35.1	0.3

ITALIAN DISHES

FOOD NAME

RAVIOLI WITH TOMATO CREAM SAUCE with heavy cream, tomatoes, basil, and Parmesan cheese

RICOTTA-STUFFED RAVIOLI WITH WALNUT SAUCE with heavy cream, walnuts, and Parmesan cheese

RIGATONI, BAKED rigatoni pasta with Italian sausage, tomatoes, basil, and mozzarella and Parmesan cheeses

RIGATONI WITH TOMATO SAUCE rigatoni pasta with tomatoes, olive oil, basil, garlic, onion, and Romano cheese

RISOTTO MILANESE with rice, saffron, chicken stock, white wine, and Parmesan cheese

RISOTTO WITH ASPARAGUS with rice, pancetta, asparagus, and white wine

RISOTTO WITH CORN AND SWEET PEPPER with rice, pancetta, corn, and peppers

RISOTTO WITH HAM, PINE NUTS, AND BASIL with rice, ham, pine nuts, basil, chicken stock and Parmesan cheese

RISOTTO WITH MUSHROOMS IN RED WINE with rice, pancetta, mushrooms, butter, onions, garlic, chicken stock, parsley, red wine, and Parmesan cheese

RISOTTO WITH MUSHROOMS IN WHITE WINE with rice, fresh mushrooms, white wine, chicken stock, and Parmesan cheese

RISOTTO WITH SAUSAGE with rice, Italian sausage and white wine

RISOTTO WITH SHRIMP with rice, shrimp, white wine, tomatoes, and fish stock

RISOTTO WITH SPINACH with rice, scallions, parsley, spinach, chicken stock, and Parmesan cheese

SPAGHETTI AND MEATBALLS spaghetti pasta with ground beef chuck, Parmesan cheese, tomatoes and red wine

Serving Size	Calories	Fat (g)	Sodium (mg)	Carbohydrate (g)	Cholesterol (mg)	Fiber (g)
1¼ cups	587.1	20.9	**1001.1**	74.4	56	1.61
1¼ cups	**1207.4**	**75.9**	875.7	87.7	193.7	0.7
1¾ cups	524.8	31.8	**1123.6**	27.8	91.7	0.8
1¼ cups	502.3	15.9	645.9	64.2	38.7	1.04
1¼ cups	427.3	14.7	**1297.3**	48.4	35.5	0.1
1½ cups	343.2	11.8	**1209**	35.1	33.3	0.3
1¾ cups	486.9	17.2	**1750**	54.3	45.2	0.5
1¼ cups	628.5	28.8	**1523.3**	62.6	40.1	0.5
1½ cups	477.7	18.3	**1565.6**	41.3	49.1	0.5
1½ cups	554.1	22.9	**1769.4**	50.7	49	0.6
1½ cups	499	25.1	**1413.8**	39.1	67	0.1
1½ cups	409.7	13.5	458.1	42.3	132.2	0.5
1½ cups	470.9	20.2	**1565**	47.3	49	0.4
1½ cups	717.9	28	699.3	57.4	165.8	0.8

ITALIAN DISHES

FOOD NAME

SPAGHETTI CARBONARA   spaghetti pasta with pancetta, eggs, heavy cream, and Parmesan cheese
SPAGHETTI WITH PANCETTA   *Bucatini Amatriciana*   with spaghetti pasta, tomatoes, pancetta and Parmesan cheese
SPAGHETTINI WITH GARLIC AND PEPPER   spaghettini pasta with garlic, pepper and Romano cheese
SPAGHETTINI WITH SWEET PEPPERS, OLIVES, AND CAPERS   spaghettini pasta with Romano and Parmesan cheeses, sweet peppers, olives, and capers
SPINACH FETTUCCINE WITH ASPARAGUS AND BACON   with spinach fettuccine pasta, asparagus, bacon, chicken stock, basil, and tomatoes
SPINACH LASAGNE WITH SPINACH AND RICOTTA   spinach lasagne with eggs, spinach, ricotta, Parmesan and mozzarella cheeses, and tomato sauce
SPINACH TORTELLINI SALAD WITH FRESH SPINACH AND PESTO   with spinach tortellini, red onion, pine nuts, and Gorgonzola
TAGLIARINI WITH FOUR CHEESES   tagliarini pasta with Fontina, Gorgonzola, Bel Paese, and Parmesan cheese
TAGLIARINI WITH ONION SAUCE   tagliarini pasta with tomatoes, onions, herbs, and Romano cheeses
SPINACH AND EGG PASTA WITH MUSHROOMS   with mushrooms, peas, prosciutto and Parmesan cheese
ZITI BAKED WITH RICOTTA CHEESE   ziti pasta with eggs, ricotta, Parmesan and mozzarella cheeses, and marinara sauce
ZITI WITH GREEN AND RED PEPPERS   ziti pasta with green and red peppers, tomatoes, basil, parsley, and Romano cheese

Serving Size	Calories	Fat (g)	Sodium (mg)	Carbohydrate (g)	Cholesterol (mg)	Fiber (g)
1¼ cups	668.6	33	**1065.2**	55.2	266.4	0
1¼ cups	392.8	10	296.1	45.6	11.6	0.6
¾ cup	374.7	16.4	330.1	42.5	2.1	.03
1½ cups	763.6	30.8	**1183.2**	82.6	48	0.8
1¼ cups	419.4	5.6	762.1	58.4	10.6	1
1½ cups	638	32.5	**1511.8**	51.1	212.5	1.8
1 cup	468.1	24.5	382.4	44.9	12.9	0.4
1 cup	638.4	32.7	818.1	47.5	103	.06
1¼ cups	417.7	13.2	431.8	57.8	16.6	1
1½ cups	400.5	9.9	**1080.1**	50.6	30.4	0.7
1¾ cups	779	31.5	**1930.3**	81.8	186.2	2.4
1½ cups	432	8.3	404.9	72	5.8	1.2

ITALIAN DISHES

FOOD NAME

ZITI WITH SUMMER SAUCE ziti pasta with zucchini, red bell peppers, tomatoes, and Provolone cheese

Seafood Dishes
Lowest Fat: *Stuffed Clams Oreganata—12.6 g fat, 309.6 calories*
Highest Fat: *Fried Seafood—133.9 g fat, 1680.6 calories*

BURRIDA fish stew with anchovies, clam juice, and tomatoes

COLD CALAMARI SALAD with squid, red onion, celery, tomatoes, garlic, lime juice, salt, pepper, olive oil, and parsley

CLAMS IN BRODO clams with olive oil, garlic, white wine, and parsley

CLAMS, STUFFED, OREGANATA clams with Parmesan cheese and marinara sauce

FISH STEW *Cioppino* with porcini mushrooms, tomatoes, fish fillets, shrimp, scallops, and lobster tails

LOBSTER FRA DIAVOLO lobster with hot pepper, marinara sauce, and spaghettini

OYSTERS BAKED WITH SPINACH AND SAMBUCA oysters with heavy cream, Parmesan cheese, bread crumbs, and Sambuca

SALMON STEAKS WITH LEMON-CAPER BUTTER salmon steaks with parsley, garlic, and olive oil

SEAFOOD, FRIED *Fritto Misto di Mare* with smelts, shrimp, scallops, cod, squid, and garlic anchovy sauce

SHRIMP OREGANATA WITH BLACK PEPPER shell-on shrimp fried in butter, olive oil, garlic, white wine, pepper, and oregano

SHRIMP SCAMPI Shrimp with olive oil, oregano, garlic, and lemon

SOLE OREGANATA filet of sole with white wine, clam juice, olive oil, and tomatoes

Serving Size	Calories	Fat (g)	Sodium (mg)	Carbohydrate (g)	Cholesterol (mg)	Fiber (g)
1½ cups	401.7	11.3	524.5	57.7	17.1	1.2
2 cups	401	12.9	428.3	5.2	131.3	0.5
¾ cup	375.1	21.6	**872.8**	17.1	386.8	.57
10 oz	376.6	27.1	71.8	5.9	40.1	.05
4 clams	309.6	12.6	773.6	20.4	56.6	0.48
2½ cups	702.5	19.9	**1039.3**	29.7	347.5	0.9
8 oz (½ lobster or 2 tails)	949	39.7	**2246.1**	65.1	**378.7**	4.1
6 oysters	673.2	21	875.7	19.5	101.4	0.2
1 8-oz steak	439.2	30.2	599	0.6	151	.02
14 oz	**1680.6**	**133.9**	**1226.1**	38.6	276.5	0.3
8 oz (8 to 10 shrimp)	528.6	25.1	540.5	27.4	251.6	.07
6 oz (4 shrimp)	420.8	30	519.8	2.2	260	.03
1 8-oz fillet	363.4	15.7	451.2	9	116.8	0.4

ITALIAN DISHES

FOOD NAME

SWORDFISH IN MARINARA SAUCE   swordfish with bread crumbs, Romano cheese, and oregano

SWORDFISH, STUFFED, SICILIAN-STYLE   swordfish with bread crumbs, prosciutto, currants, and mint

TUNA, GRILLED, WITH TOMATO-CAPER SAUCE   tuna grilled with tomato sauce, capers, garlic, oregano, parsley, and olive oil

TROUT STUFFED WITH PROSCIUTTO AND BREAD CRUMBS

Desserts
Lowest Fat: Biscotti—1 g fat, 108 calories
Highest Fat: Cannoli with Hazelnut Cream—51.2 g fat, 659 calories

BAKED APPLES   apples baked with sugar, currants, walnuts, butter, and Chianti

BISCOTTI (plain)   with flour, sugar, eggs, milk, cream, and vanilla

BISCUIT TORTONI   ice cream with almonds, macaroons, and dark rum

CANNOLI WITH HAZELNUT CREAM   cannoli pastry with heavy cream, sugar, vanilla, and pistachio nuts

CHEESECAKE, ITALIAN-STYLE   with golden raisins, Marsala, ricotta cheese, and pine nuts

COFFEE GRANITÀ   *Granità di Caffe*   with espresso, heavy cream, and apricot brandy

ICE CREAM, ITALIAN   *Spumoni*   with milk, eggs, sugar, vanilla, almonds, cream, cherries, candied fruit, and light rum

RISOTTO PUDDING   with Arborio rice, golden raisins, strawberries, blueberries, and cream

TIRAMISÙ   with ladyfingers, espresso, brandy, marscapone cheese, and cocoa powder

Serving Size	Calories	Fat (g)	Sodium (mg)	Carbohydrate (g)	Cholesterol (mg)	Fiber (g)
6 oz	387.8	20.3	**1395.4**	19.6	64	1.94
6 oz	280.5	13.8	626.9	8.7	57.6	0.2
8 oz	481.1	22.8	511.5	6.2	98	0.7
1 1-pound trout	762.1	37.7	354.9	3.8	265.2	.03
1 8-oz apple	227	6	46	35.4	10.3	1.2
2 biscotti	108	1	10	22.8	27.2	.04
3 oz	455	42	39	11.9	108.7	0.6
1 4-oz cannoli	**659**	**51.2**	32.5	89.9	108.7	0.4
4 oz	495	30	215	37	277.2	0.1
10 oz	183	11	15	19.8	40.8	0
½ cup	229.8	12.7	30	25.1	123.3	0.1
1¼ cups	585	16	300	92.4	49.1	0.8
⅔ cup	433	36	297	16	255	.04

ITALIAN DISHES

FOOD NAME

TRIFLE, ITALIAN *Zuppa Inglese* with almonds, lemon, sweet vermouth, dark rum, ladyfingers, and apricot preserves
ZABAGLIONE with Marsala wine or sherry, egg yolks, and sugar

Serving Size	Calories	Fat (g)	Sodium (mg)	Carbohydrate (g)	Cholesterol (mg)	Fiber (g)
⅔ cup	393	20	207	40.8	147	0.6
¼ cup	151	8	15	9.7	408	0

Japanese Cuisine

The good news is that Japanese cuisine is wonderfully low in fat; the bad news is that many dishes, teriyaki for example, are loaded with sodium, so individuals monitoring their salt intake or suffering from high blood pressure need to order cautiously. When eating sushi, use soy sauce (very high in sodium) sparingly. In addition, remember that shellfish is relatively high in cholesterol, and some fish, such as eel and roe, are fatty. As always, fried dishes, such as tempura, are not the best choice. With these few exceptions, feel free to enjoy almost anything listed on a Japanese menu. For those who have avoided Japanese restaurants because they don't like the idea of eating raw fish, don't forget that typical Japanese menus also feature delicious broiled fish dishes, boiled meat and vegetables, noodle dishes, and vegetarian options as well. There are delicious broths, such as miso, and a variety of low-fat noodles. This is perhaps the most healthy cuisine in the world. Possibly this explains why Japanese restaurants have skyrocketed in popularity over the last decade.

JAPANESE DISHES

FOOD NAME

Appetizers, Salads, and Vegetables
Lowest Fat: Vegetable Salad—12.8 g fat, 141.3 calories
Highest Fat: Tempura—56.9 g fat, 709.7 calories

TEMPURA, VEGETABLE   Deep-fried acorn squash, mushrooms, lotus root, carrot, green pepper, and sweet potato

TOFU SALAD WITH SESAME DRESSING   bean curd with Romaine lettuce, cucumber, orange, watercress, oil, vinegar, soy sauce, mustard, sesame seeds, and garlic

VEGETABLE SALAD   with mixed salad greens, red cabbage, cucumber, radishes, carrots, oil, vinegar, sherry, sesame seeds, lemon juice, and soy sauce

Soups
Lowest Fat: Clear Mushroom Soup—0.7 g fat, 39.1 calories
Highest Fat: Clear Tofu Flower Soup—3.5 g fat, 97.3 calories

CLEAR MUSHROOM SOUP   *Kinko no suimono*   with white radish, shiitake mushrooms, white mushrooms, kelp, bonito flakes, and soy sauce

MISO SOUP   *Miso-Shiru*   with wakame seaweed, potatoes, and dashi

CLEAR TOFU FLOWER SOUP   with bean curd, carrot, green beans, dashi, salt, and soy sauce

Sashimi (Raw Seafood)
Lowest Fat: Scallops—0.4 g fat, 50.3 calories
Highest Fat: Mackerel—7.9 g fat, 116.6 calories

EEL

MACKEREL

SALMON

SCALLOPS

SHARK

Serving Size	Calories	Fat (g)	Sodium (mg)	Carbohydrate (g)	Cholesterol (mg)	Fiber (g)
6 oz (approx. 4-6 pieces)	**709.7**	**56.9**	37.7	34.9	91.3	1
1 cup	178.7	15.3	538.4	5	0	0.4
1¼ cups	141.3	12.8	274.3	6.2	0	0.8
1¼ cups	39.1	0.7	**909**	4.5	0	1.1
1¼ cups	54.1	0.9	363.1	6.5	0	0.6
1¼ cups	97.3	3.5	714.9	4.4	0	0.4
1 2-oz roll	104.5	6.6	28.8	0	71.7	0
1 2-oz roll	**116.6**	**7.9**	50.9	0	40.2	0
1 2-oz roll	81.1	3.6	24.8	0	31.5	0
1 2-oz roll	50.3	0.4	91.8	1.3	18.8	0
1 2-oz roll	74.4	2.6	44.9	0	28.8	0

JAPANESE DISHES

FOOD NAME

SHRIMP

SQUID

TUNA

WHITEFISH

YELLOWTAIL

Cone Sushi (with rice and filling in a seaweed wrapper)
Lowest Fat: *Hand-wrapped Sushi with Cucumber—0.2 g fat, 30.8 calories*
Highest Fat: *Hand-wrapped Sushi with Avocado—6.3 g fat, 91.4 calories*

CONE SUSHI WITH AVOCADO

CONE SUSHI WITH CRAB

CONE SUSHI WITH CUCUMBER

CONE SUSHI WITH EGG

CONE SUSHI WITH SALMON ROE

CONE SUSHI WITH SMOKED SALMON

Roll Sushi (rice and fillings rolled in seaweed and sliced into bite-sized pieces)
Lowest Fat: *Kappa-Maki—0.1 g fat, 56.7 calories*
Highest Fat: *Alaskan Roll—4.8 g fat, 96.2 calories*

ALASKAN ROLL   with salmon, avocado, and cucumber

CALIFORNIA ROLL   with crab, avocado, and cucumber

FUTO-MAKI   with egg, cucumber, and crab

KAPPA-MAKI   with cucumber

NORI-MAKI   with salmon

Serving Size	Calories	Fat (g)	Sodium (mg)	Carbohydrate (g)	Cholesterol (mg)	Fiber (g)
1 2-oz roll	60.3	1	84.4	0.5	87.1	0
1 2-oz roll	99.8	4.3	174.2	4.4	148.1	0
1 2-oz roll	104.5	3.6	28.8	0	28.1	0
1 2-oz roll	76.4	3.3	28.8	0	34.2	0
1 2-oz roll	92.5	3.6	49.6	0	36.9	0
1 2-oz cone	**91.4**	**6.3**	18.5	8	0	1
1 2-oz cone	74.2	0.5	490.6	5.0	23.5	0.1
1 2-oz cone	30.8	0.2	15.5	6.8	0	0.5
1 2-oz cone	105.6	5.7	83.3	5.6	274	0.1
1 2-oz cone	186.6	3.7	814.3	5.8	212	0.1
1 2-oz cone	127.1	5.4	**910.9**	5	21.6	0.1
1 2-oz roll	**96.2**	**4.8**	27.6	6.7	14.1	0.6
1 2-oz roll	74.1	3.3	158.7	6.7	7	0.6
1 2-oz roll	80.4	2.5	255.3	5.4	120.1	0.2
1 2-oz roll	38.6	0.1	261.4	12.3	0	.08
1 2-oz roll	55	0.7	545.3	.8.8	24.8	0

JAPANESE DISHES

FOOD NAME

TEKKA-MAKI with tuna

Main Dishes
Lowest Fat: *Grilled Prawns in the Shell—1 g fat, 77.5 calories*
Highest Fat: *Teriyaki Beef—24.8 g fat, 386.7 calories*

CHICKEN PATTIES *Noshidori* with chicken, egg, sugar, sake, ginger juice, and soy sauce

MARINATED SALMON NANBAN *Wakasagi no nanban-zuke* with marinated salmon fillets, onions, carrot, green peppers, lemon, oil, parsley, flour, sugar, salt, soy sauce, vinegar, and chile peppers

CHICKEN DONBURI *Oyako Donburi* with chicken, rice, sugar, soy sauce, dashi, onions, sake, and eggs

MARBLED EGGS *Ganseki tamago* Hard-boiled eggs seasoned with sake and sugar

PRAWNS IN THE SHELL *Ebi no onigara yaki* grilled shrimp with sake and salt

RARE BEEF *Gyuniku no tataki* beef lightly grilled, with ginger, garlic, shallots, shiso leaves, oil, soy, and daikon

SALMON RICE *Sake gohan* Salmon with sesame, ginger, and green shiso

SOBA NOODLES WITH BEAN SPROUTS AND CARROTS buckwheat noodles with bean sprouts and carrots

SOBA NOODLES WITH EGG TOPPING buckwheat noodles with sugar, salt, and oil

SOBA NOODLES WITH STIR-FRIED PORK buckwheat noodles with pork, sugar, ginger, scallions, cornstarch, oil, sake, mirin, and soy sauce

SOBA NOODLES WITH STEAMED CHICKEN buckwheat noodles, steamed chicken, red chilies, sake, and soy sauce

Serving Size	Calories	Fat (g)	Sodium (mg)	Carbohydrate (g)	Cholesterol (mg)	Fiber (g)
1 2-oz roll	60.7	0.3	262.9	12.2	1.5	0
1 5-oz patty	323.4	16.6	546.5	2.8	153	0
1 6-oz fillet	289.0	11.1	859.4	9.4	94	0.4
1½ cups	577.3	15	556.9	73.4	274.5	0.3
1 oz	57.7	3.7	35.8	2.3	182.3	0
2 large shrimp (2 oz)	77.5	1	322.1	0.5	86.7	0
6 oz	348.3	18.9	335.2	1.4	103.9	0.1
1½ cups	587.1	12.3	308.1	80.2	78.3	0.5
two cups	403.0	1.6	**1080.5**	87.2	0	4.4
2 cups	488	8.6	**1038.1**	86.9	274	4
2 cups	593.3	14.2	**1506.2**	89.8	65.8	4
2 cups	570.5	9.7	**1408.4**	87.4	61.3	4

JAPANESE DISHES

FOOD NAME

SUKIYAKI   with beef, tofu, shiitake mushrooms, onions, scallions, spinach, oil, glass noodles, sugar, sake, mirin, and soy sauce
TERIYAKI, BEEF   *beef marinated in Teriyaki Sauce*
TERIYAKI, CHICKEN   *Tori no teriyaki*   chicken marinated in Teriyaki Sauce
TERIYAKI, SALMON   *Sake no teriyaki*   salmon marinated in Teriyaki Sauce
TERIYAKI, SHRIMP   *Ebi no teriyaki*   shrimp marinated in Teriyaki Sauce (see page 148)

Desserts

Lowest Fat: *Japanese Pancakes with Sweet Bean Paste Filling—5.6 g fat, 377.2 calories*
Highest Fat: *Green Tea Ice Cream—12.7 g fat, 184.5 calories*

GREEN TEA ICE CREAM   with cream, milk, green tea and vanilla
JAPANESE PANCAKES WITH SWEET BEAN PASTE FILLING   *Dorayaki*   with eggs, flour, sugar, honey, mirin, and azuki beans

Basics

BEAN CURD   *Tofu*   made from soy beans
GINGER ROOT   *Shoga*
JAPANESE STEAK SAUCE   with onion, butter, soy, chili sauce, sake, mustard, and pepper
ORIENTAL RICE   with short or medium-grain white rice
RICE FOR SUSHI   rice with vinegar, sugar and salt
SAKE   rice wine
SEAWEED   *Nori*
SOBA NOODLES   *Soba*   with buckwheat flour and light wheat flour

Serving Size	Calories	Fat (g)	Sodium (mg)	Carbohydrate (g)	Cholesterol (mg)	Fiber (g)
2 cups	436.5	18.3	**1703.1**	19.1	92.3	0.7
6 oz	**386.7**	**24.8**	1096.4	6.0	98	0
6 oz	402.8	20.1	822.8	4.0	138.0	0
6 oz	265.7	10.8	417.2	3.4	94.0	0
6 oz	202.9	7	553.1	4.1	216.7	0
½ cup	**184.5**	**12.7**	36.1	14.3	148	0
1 double-layer pancake	377.2	5.6	50.5	64.5	109.6	1.3
6 oz	123.4	7.2	606.8	4.1	0	0.2
1 oz	8.0	0.2	2	1.8	0	0.2
1 oz	167.3	12.1	**1102**	9.8	31	0.3
1 cup cooked	118	0.3	1.7	26.2	0	0.1
1 cup cooked	284.7	0.5	890	65.4	0	0.1
1 oz	97	0	1	11.5	0	0
1 oz	10	0.1	14	1.4	0	0.1
1 cup	192	0.4	449	42.5	0	2

JAPANESE DISHES

FOOD NAME

SOY SAUCE *Shoyu* from soy beans, wheat, and salt
TEMPURA SAUCE with soy sauce, beef broth, brown sugar, sake, daikon, and ginger
TERIYAKI SAUCE with soy sauce, mirin, ginger, and garlic
WAKAME Sea vegetable
WASABI green horseradish

Serving Size	Calories	Fat (g)	Sodium (mg)	Carbohydrate (g)	Cholesterol (mg)	Fiber (g)
2 tblsp	22	0	**2058**	3	0	0
½ cup	60.4	0.2	**1633.4**	7.9	0	0
2 tblsp	84.6	0	**1373**	11	0	0
1 oz	13	0.2	247	2.6	0	0.2
½ teaspoon	7.9	0	2	1.6	0	0

Mexican Cuisine

A Mexican meal can be either high in fat or wonderfully healthy, depending on how it is prepared and served. Rice, beans, and corn—three staples in Mexican cuisine—are nutritious and low in fat. However, when these staples are cooked with lard and cheese, the saturated fat and cholesterol contents rise considerably. Make sure refried beans are fried in vegetable oil rather than lard, and choose soft rather than hard (deep-fried) tortillas. Salsa is an excellent substitute for high-fat guacamole and sour cream. Made entirely of vegetables (typically tomatoes, onions, chilies, and cilantro), salsa contains no saturated fat. Just make sure your enthusiasm for this low-fat treat doesn't lead you to overdo it on the nacho chips! Keep meat and cheese to a minimum, as these are high-fat foods, and choose items that are grilled or broiled rather than fried. A bean burrito, without cheese, in a flour tortilla with as much salsa as you like is a delicious alternative to cheese-laden nachos or fried tacos with meat. When cooking Mexican food at home, substitute no-fat or low-fat cheese for the high-fat cheeses traditionally served with Mexican dishes. Substituting ground turkey for ground beef will also cut down on the amount of fat contained in many popular dishes. Try Mexican-style rice instead of chips as a side dish. Margaritas and daiquiris are packed with sugar and should therefore be taken in moderation. Be wary of opting for a fancy coffee instead of dessert—you may not be doing yourself a favor. Any coffee drink described as "creamy" is going to add fat calories to your meal. A good choice is Spanish coffee, served with only a dollop of coffee liqueur. Don't add extra sugar or cream. If you have dessert, remember to skip the whipped cream and share the treat with a friend.

MEXICAN DISHES

FOOD NAME

Appetizers
Lowest Fat: *Jicama Appetizer—0 g fat, 71 calories*
Highest Fat: *Nachos with Refried Beans—43 g fat, 738.7 calories*

CHEESE TOSTADAS *Tostadas de Harina con Queso* flour tortilla with Cheddar cheese and green chilies

FISH APPETIZER, ACAPULCO STYLE *Seviche de Acapulco* raw fish fillets marinated in citrus juice with chilies and tomatoes

GRILLED CHEESE AND TORTILLAS *Queso al Horno* with melted Monterey Jack cheese, served on corn tortillas with chile sauce

JICAMA APPETIZER *Jicama Fresca* crisp root vegetable with chili powder and lime

NACHOS deep-fried corn tortilla chips with Cheddar cheese and jalapeños

NACHOS WITH REFRIED BEANS tortilla chips with shredded Cheddar and Monterey Jack cheeses, refried beans, tomatoes, onions, olives, salsa, and sour cream

NACHOS WITH REFRIED BEANS AND GROUND BEEF tortilla chips with refried beans, ground beef, onion, black olives, tortilla chips, green chilies, and shredded Cheddar cheese

PEANUTS, OAXACAN *Cacahuetes* salted peanuts tossed with chilies, garlic, and olive oil

QUESADILLAS fried corn tortillas filled with chilies and Monterey Jack cheese

REFRIED BEAN DIP *Aperitivo de Frijoles Refritos* with Cheddar cheese and taco sauce

TOSTADA BITES, OAXACAN corn tortillas with black bean and mole sauce

Serving Size	Calories	Fat (g)	Sodium (mg)	Carbohydrate (g)	Cholesterol (mg)	Fiber (g)
⅛ tortilla (1 oz)	61	4	78	2.5	13.3	0.1
⅔ cup	140	7	626	5.9	24	0.2
¼ tortilla (2 pieces)	52	3	5	12.8	10	0.1
4 oz	71	0	**1339**	16.3	0	0.6
1 oz	194.4	12.7	70.6	16.6	12	0.4
6 oz	**738.7**	**43**	**1122.9**	7.5	34.2	5.1
1½ cups	364.4	21.9	583	28.8	46.5	4.9
¼ cup	249.5	21.5	133.2	9.4	0	1.2
one 9-inch quesadilla	223.2	14	222.5	14	39.9	0.4
⅓ cup	535	11.2	695	68.9	60.4	3
6 tortillas chips, each with 1 tblsp. sauce	468	18	444	86.4	12	1.2

MEXICAN DISHES

FOOD NAME

Breads
Lowest Fat: Fried Bread—1 g fat, 47 calories
Highest Fat: Corn Bread—29 g fat, 468 calories

CORNBREAD *Pastel de Elote* made with corn meal, chilies, and Monterey Jack and Cheddar cheeses

"PANTS" BISCUITS *Calzones* with flour, milk, sugar, and cinnamon

PUFF PASTRY ROLLS *Hojaldre* paper-thin pastry rolled with sugar and cinnamon

PUFFY FRIED BREAD *Sopapillas* with flour, sugar, shortening, and milk

SWEET BUNS *Pan Dulce* with flour, sugar, shortening, milk, and cinnamon

THREE KINGS' BREAD *Rosca de Los Reyes* yeast bread filled with raisins, walnuts, candied cherries, and orange and lemon peel

Soups
Lowest Fat: Corn Gazpacho—3 g fat, 164 calories
Highest Fat: Tripe and Hominy Soup—62.5 g fat, 909 calories

ASPARAGUS SOUP WITH CREAM CHEESE *Caldo de Esparrago con Queso* with asparagus, cream cheese, chicken broth

BLACK BEAN SOUP *Sopa de Frijoles Negros* with black beans, butter, ham, onions, celery, carrots, garlic, and flour

CORN GAZPACHO with corn, red peppers, cucumber, and dill

CORN SOUP *Sopa Sonorense* chicken broth with corn, green peppers, corn, and chili powder

GAZPACHO WITH AVOCADO with avocado, cucumber, onion, olive oil, oregano, vinegar, and tomato juice

MEATBALL SOUP, MEXICAN STYLE *Sopa de Albondigas* with meatballs, pine nuts and Sherry

Serving Size	Calories	Fat (g)	Sodium (mg)	Carbohydrate (g)	Cholesterol (mg)	Fiber (g)
6 oz slice	**468**	**29**	397	54.5	171.2	0.6
1 biscuit	64	3	77	8.9	0.8	0
1 small pastry	43.9	2.9	50.2	4	7.8	0
1 pastry	47	1	107	8	0.9	0
1 bun	215	8	250	31.9	64.6	0.1
one 3-oz wedge	302.8	12.7	195.5	34.4	60	0.4
1 cup	131	11	935	2.4	31.7	0.2
1 cup	203	4.6	71	30.3	10.6	0.2
1 cup	164	3	563	24.5	10.3	1
1 cup	186	15	877	7.9	49.3	0.6
1 cup	130	10	327	11.4	0	0.8
1 cup	278	22	782	7.3	73.1	0.2

MEXICAN DISHES

FOOD NAME

PORK AND HOMINY SOUP *Pozole* with pork hocks, hominy, tomatoes, and onions

RICE SOUP WITH EGGS *Sopa de Arroz con Huevos* with rice, chicken broth, shortening, tomatoes, garlic, chilies, and cilantro

TRIPE AND HOMINY SOUP *Menudo* with tripe, veal, garlic, onion, cilantro, chili powder, and scallions

Salads
Lowest Fat: Kidney Bean Salad—11 g fat, 108 calories
Highest Fat: Beef Tongue and Vegetable Salad—67 g fat, 885 calories

BEEF TONGUE AND VEGETABLE SALAD *Salpicon* beef tongue with carrots, turnips, and potatoes in vinaigrette

CHRISTMAS EVE SALAD *Ensalada de Nochebuena* with beets, oranges, apples, bananas, pineapple, and peanuts

KIDNEY BEAN SALAD *Ensalada de Frijoles* with kidney beans, celery, walnuts, and sweet pickles

MARINATED BEEF SALAD *Carne a la Vinegreta* with beef, onions, capers, and parsley in vinaigrette

PICO DE GALLO WITH ORANGE *Pico de Gallo Anaranjado* with chopped orange, cucumber, onion, pepper, and jicama on Romaine leaves

PICO DE GALLO WITH JICAMA *Pico de Gallo con Jicama* with Jicama, chopped pepper, onion and cucumber

SHRIMP SALAD IN AVOCADO HALVES *Ensalata de Camaron con Aguacate*

TOPOPO SALAD with Topopo (see page 168), chili powder, tomatoes, Romano cheese, peas, scallions, lettuce, oil, and vinegar

Serving Size	Calories	Fat (g)	Sodium (mg)	Carbohydrate (g)	Cholesterol (mg)	Fiber (g)
1 cup	130.5	8.5	599	7.7	18.6	1.3
1 cup	246	3.5	378.5	31.5	137.5	0.3
1 cup	**454.5**	**31.2**	599.3	6	120.9	0.8
1½ cups	**885**	**67**	622	40.3	222.4	2.8
2 cups	491	23	481	59.1	4.3	2.9
4 oz	108	11	501	12.8	0	1.1
1 cup	535	46	409	2.7	104.3	0.1
1½ cups	151	14	256	7.1	0	0.7
1 cup	202	14	510	19.5	0	1
7 oz of salad in a 3-oz avocado half	315	22	490	25	120	3
1 cup	327	28	519	17.5	0	2.6

MEXICAN DISHES

FOOD NAME

Beef & Pork Dishes
Lowest Fat: Beef Fajita—6.3 g fat, 129.8 calories
Highest Fat: Macaroni and Chorizo Sausage "Dry Soup"—56 g fat, 785.6 calories

BARBECUED BEEFSTEAK, MEXICAN STYLE *Bistec de Jalisco* beef with fresh orange juice

BURRITO, BEEF AND BEAN *Burrito de Frijoles y Carne* lean ground beef and refried beans in a flour tortilla

CARNE ASADA sliced grilled beef and pork with green peppers and fried bananas

CARNITAS pork shoulder with salt, oregano, onions, cumin, and carrots

CHALUPA "little boat" of fried dough filled with pork and topped with Chile-Tomato Sauce (see page 174)

CHILE VERDE beef and pork with chilies and peppers

CHILIES STUFFED WITH WALNUTS *Chiles en Nogada* with pork, tomato, apple, pear, banana, and walnuts

CHIMICHANGA fried flour tortillas filled with ground beef, Cheddar cheese, shredded lettuce, and onions

"DRY SOUP," MACARONI AND CHORIZO SAUSAGE *Sopa Seca de Macarron y Chorizo* casserole of noodles and chorizo with Monterey Jack cheese

"DRY SOUP," RICE AND CHORIZO SAUSAGE *Sopa Seca de Arroz y Chorizo* casserole of rice and chorizo sausage with onions and tomato puree

"DRY SOUP," RICE WITH PEAS AND HAM *Sopa Seca de Arroz con Chicaros y Jamón* with rice, peas, ham, onions, garlic, tomatoes, chicken broth, chilies, parsley, and green olives with pimientos

Serving Size	Calories	Fat (g)	Sodium (mg)	Carbohydrate (g)	Cholesterol (mg)	Fiber (g)
6 oz	225	17	169	1	59	0
one 4-oz burrito	343.6	21.1	330.8	21.6	64	2.6
9 oz	**756**	**56**	929.5	25	135	1
6 oz	165.4	18	207.8	1.5	28.3	0.1
one 3-oz chalupa	189.5	16	339	9	35	0.1
12 oz	**759**	**56**	332.5	16.5	160	2
one 3½-oz stuffed chile	230	17.3	153	11.3	36.5	1
one 4-oz chimichanga	147.5	10	126	7.5	27	0.2
1¼ cups	**785.6**	**56**	**1939.2**	**85.6**	0	1.4
2 cups	690.3	28.2	**1284.1**	82.5	164.5	2.6
2 cups	449	9	1670.5	72	43	1.6

MEXICAN DISHES

FOOD NAME

ENCHILADAS, BEEF AND BEAN *Enchilada de Res y Frijoles Refritos* corn tortillas filled with ground beef, refried beans, and olives, topped with Chile-Tomato Sauce (see page 174) and Cheddar cheese

ENCHILADAS, CHORIZO SAUSAGE *Enchilada de Chorizo* corn tortillas filled with chorizo sausage, topped with Chile-Tomato Sauce (see page 174), Monterey Jack and Cheddar cheeses, and Guacamole (see page 174)

ENCHILADAS, FOLDED PORK *Enchilada de Puerco Dobladas* with Chile-Tomato Sauce (page 174), and Monterey Jack cheese

ENCHILADAS, ROLLED BEEF *Enchiladas de Res Enrolladas* corn tortillas filled with ground beef and chile sauce

FAJITA, BEEF steak with onions, peppers, and spices on a flour tortilla

FLAUTAS WITH BEEF fried, flute-shaped tacos with ground beef, onion, and Red Chile Sauce (see page 176)

FLAUTAS WITH CHORIZO SAUSAGE fried, flute-shaped taco with ground beef, ground pork, onion, chile, vinegar and Chile-Tomato Sauce (see page 174)

FLAUTAS WITH PORK fried, flute-shaped tacos with shredded pork, onions, jalapeños, olives, and Red Chile Sauce (see page 176)

GARNACHES WITH BEEF fried dough cakes filled with beef and Cheddar cheese

GARNACHES WITH PORK with Cheddar cheese, onion, chilies, raisins, olives, and Red Chile Sauce (see page 176)

GORDITAS "fat little" dough cakes with chorizo sausage and Monterey Jack cheese

POT ROAST, MEXICAN STYLE braised beef brisket with carrots, tomatoes, raisins, and olives

Serving Size	Calories	Fat (g)	Sodium (mg)	Carbohydrate (g)	Cholesterol (mg)	Fiber (g)
1 6-oz enchilada	159.4	11.1	309.3	8.5	27	0.9
1 4-oz enchilada	413.8	30	676.9	20	59.3	0.9
1 4-oz enchilada	198.1	12.5	209.9	13.6	17.8	0.5
1 4-oz enchilada	310	23	435.7	15.3	41.3	0.4
1 5-oz fajita	129.8	6.3	192.6	11.6	14.9	0.4
1 5-oz flauta	293	16	98	28	32	0.7
1 5-oz flauta	347.5	18.8	386.3	35	34.4	0.9
1 5-oz flauta	375.1	22.5	162.7	29.1	37.5	0.5
1 4-oz garnache	357	31	576	18	65	0.5
1 4-oz garnache	383.5	31.5	606	19	63	0.6
2 2-oz gorditas	296	26	803	25	6	1.6
12 oz	568.6	38.1	**458.4**	21.1	122.5	1.9

MEXICAN DISHES

FOOD NAME

STEAK SANDWICH *El Pepito* barbecued steak on roll with refried beans and guacamole

TACO, BEEF *Taco de Carne Asada* steak and spices in a deep-fried corn tortilla shell

TACO SALAD ground beef, onions, pinto beans, tomatoes, olives, avocado, Cheddar cheese and lettuce in a deep-fried flour tortilla

TOSTADAS WITH BEEF *Tostadas de Res* with beef, corn tortillas, refried beans, Cheddar cheese, lettuce, and tomatoes

TOSTADAS WITH PORK *Tostadas de Puerco* with pork, corn tortillas, refried beans, Cheddar cheese, lettuce, and tomatoes

Chicken and Poultry Dishes
Lowest Fat: Taco, Chicken—13.1 g fat, 231.8 calories
Highest Fat: Chicken Enchiladas, Uruapán—32.7 g fat, 491.7 calories

BURRITO, CHICKEN *Burrito de Pollo* with chicken, refried beans, sour cream, avocado, tomato, watercress, and lime juice

CHONITAS turnovers with chicken, onions, raisins, olives, tomatoes and chilies

ENCHILADAS, ACAPULCO *Enchiladas de Acapulco* with diced chicken, olives, almonds, chile sauce, and Cheddar cheese

ENCHILADAS, CHICKEN PICADILLO flour tortillas filled with shredded chicken, raisins, tomatoes, almonds, and olives

ENCHILADAS WITH CHICKEN, URUAPÁN *Enchiladas de Pollo de Uruapán* corn tortilla filled with Romano and Monterey Jack cheeses and topped with sautéed chicken

FLAUTAS WITH CHICKEN fried, flute-shaped tacos with scallions, butter and pimientos

GARNACHES WITH CHICKEN masa dough cakes with chicken, scallions, pimientos, Cheddar cheese, and onion

Serving Size	Calories	Fat (g)	Sodium (mg)	Carbohydrate (g)	Cholesterol (mg)	Fiber (g)
1 6-oz sandwich	722	37	943	67	89	1.4
1 taco with 2 oz of steak	193.8	10	217.8	13.5	29.8	0.3
2 cups	827.1	50.5	423	66.2	84	5.4
1 8-oz tostada	353	26.5	471	54	22	1.7
1 8-oz tostada	367.5	27	487.5	55	21	1.8
1 6-oz burrito	262.7	14.4	355.5	165.8	50.6	2.7
1 4-oz chonita	483	32.3	614	32	62	1
1 6-oz enchilada	344.7	25.9	315.7	15.7	51.7	0.7
1 6½-oz enchilada	361.3	16.5	205.5	54.8	29.3	1.3
1 5-oz enchilada	491.7	32.7	530.7	52.3	95	0.6
1 3-oz flauta	316	19	132	29	29	0.8
1 4-oz garnache	351	27	608	17	62	0.6

MEXICAN DISHES

FOOD NAME

TACO, CHICKEN *Taco de Pollo* shredded breast meat with olive oil, salt, and pepper in a deep-fried corn tortilla

TOSTADAS WITH CHICKEN *Tostadas de Pollo* with corn tortillas, refried beans, Cheddar cheese, lettuce, and tomato

TOSTADAS WITH TURKEY *Tostadas de Ave* with corn tortillas, refried beans, Cheddar cheese, lettuce, and tomato

Seafood Dishes
Lowest Fat: Fish Taco—11.9 g fat, 326.4 calories
Highest Fat: Breaded Fish—27 g fat, 400 calories

BREADED FISH *Pescado Empanado* fried fish, with scallops, white wine, onion, garlic, egg, bread crumbs, and lemon juice

"DRY SOUP" WITH RICE AND SHRIMP *Sopa Seca de Arroz y Camarón* with rice, shrimp, onion, garlic, tomatoes, chicken broth, chilies, parsley, and green olives

FISH TACO *Taco de Pescado* corn tortilla with red snapper, Tabasco sauce, clove, Worcestershire sauce, and lemon juice

SEAFOOD ENCHILADA *Enchilada de Mariscos* corn tortilla filled with rice, crabmeat, scallions, and Monterey Jack cheese, topped with Red Chile Sauce (see page 176), sour cream, and black olives

SHRIMPS IN CHIPOLTE SAUCE *Camarones Enchipotlados* with large shrimp, lime juice, olive oil, onion, tomatoes, garlic, chile peppers, white wine, oregano, sea salt and pepper

SHRIMP, FRIED *Camarón Frito* large, butterflied shrimp coated with almond butter and deep-fried

TOSTADA WITH CRAB *Tostada de Cangrejo* with crab, avocado, lettuce, refried beans, and Cheddar cheese

Serving Size	Calories	Fat (g)	Sodium (mg)	Carbohydrate (g)	Cholesterol (mg)	Fiber (g)
1 3-oz taco	231.8	13.1	223.7	13.5	49	0.3
1 9-oz tostada	350	25	488	55	20	1.8
1 9-oz tostada	348	24.5	493	55	20	1.8
7 oz	**400**	**27**	**1788**	11	142	0.1
2 cups	**489.5**	16	870	63	127.7	0.6
1 5-oz taco	326.4	11.9	180.6	33.4	57.9	0.4
2 enchiladas	463.2	21.9	654	49.1	23.7	1.3
8 oz	402.6	26.8	403.3	11.0	216.7	.90
9 oz (about 9 shrimp)	446	20	341	26	325	0.4
1 7½-oz tostada	328	24.5	630	26.5	57.5	2

MEXICAN DISHES

FOOD NAME

Egg Dishes
Lowest Fat: Green Chile Enchilada Soufflé—17.5 g fat, 264 calories
Highest Fat: Chilaquiles—56 g fat, 757 calories

CACTUS OMELET *Tortilla de Huevos* with eggs, cactus meat, and chorizo sausage

CHILAQUILES fried tortilla strips with eggs, chilies, and cheese

FRIED EGGS WITH CHEESE *Huevos con Queso* eggs and cheese with butter

GREEN CHILE ENCHILADA SOUFFLÉ *Enchiladas de Chile Verde en Soufflé* with cheese and chilies baked in a tortilla-lined dish

HARD-COOKED EGGS WITH CHILE AND AVOCADO SAUCE *Huevos con Chile y Salsa de Aguacates*

HUEVOS RANCHEROS eggs fried in butter with refried beans, Cheddar cheese, chile sauce, and avocado on corn tortillas

MEXICAN OMELET *Tortilla de Huevos* with butter, green olives, and green chilies

Vegetarian Dishes
Lowest Fat: Squash Chili—4.5 g fat, 100 calories
Highest Fat: Topopo—44 g fat, 791 calories

BURRITO, VEGETARIAN burrito with zucchini, squash, and salsa

CHILE AND CHEESE SANDWICH *Chiles con Queso Seco* California chilies and Monterey Jack cheese on bread

CHILES RELLENOS chile peppers stuffed with Monterey Jack cheese, covered in egg batter and deep-fried

CHILES RELLENOS CON PICADILLO chile peppers stuffed with Monterey Jack cheese, covered in egg batter and deep-fried, with picadillo

Serving Size	Calories	Fat (g)	Sodium (mg)	Carbohydrate (g)	Cholesterol (mg)	Fiber (g)
6 oz	479.5	37	**1741**	13.5	853	1.2
6 oz	530.2	37	813	23.3	411	.95
2 eggs	296	24	560	19.6	568.6	0
4 oz	264	17.5	500.5	19	170.8	0.4
8 oz (2 eggs with sauce)	412	33.5	475	15	568	2.8
12 oz	494	37	543	63.5	289	5
1 2-egg omelet	229	19	**1216**	2	568.5	0.2
1 4-oz burrito	166.5	7.4	419	25.1	0	1.7
5 oz	422	32	150	74.5	67	8.6
1 5-oz chile	266.5	17.5	79.5	46.8	228.5	0.5
1 5-oz chile	325	21	444.5	15	265.5	0.8

MEXICAN DISHES

FOOD NAME

CHILES RELLENOS CON FRIJOLES   chile peppers stuffed with beans, tomatoes and Cheddar cheese
"DRY SOUP," RICE   *Sopa Seca de Arroz*   tomato-flavored rice casserole
"DRY SOUP," RICE WITH HEARTS OF PALM   *Arroz con Palmito*   with Rice "Dry Soup" (above), hearts of palm, and salt pork
"DRY SOUP" WITH TORTILLA   *Sopa Seca de Tortilla*   spicy, tortilla casserole with cheese and chile
EGGPLANT ACAPULCO   *Berenjena de Acapulco*   baked, with mushrooms and Romano cheese
ENCHILADAS, SONORA, WITH MASA DOUGH   *Enchiladas de Sonora con Masa*   fried flour cakes coated and filled with cheese and covered with Chile-Tomato Sauce (see page 174)
ENCHILADAS, SOUR CREAM   *Enchiladas de Jocoque*   corn tortilla filled with Cheddar cheese and sour cream
ENCHILADAS, STACKED CHEESE   *Enchiladas de Queso*   corn tortilla with chile sauce and Cheddar cheese
SOPES   flour-dough cakes fried in lard, with refried beans and Cheddar cheese
SQUASH CHILI   with red peppers, tomatoes, and kidney beans
TOPOPO   main-dish salad with corn tortillas, refried beans, avocado, shrimp, and cheese
TOSTADA WITH REFRIED BEANS   with Cheddar cheese, lettuce, and tomato on a deep-fried corn tortilla

Serving Size	Calories	Fat (g)	Sodium (mg)	Carbohydrate (g)	Cholesterol (mg)	Fiber (g)
4 oz	147	14.5	306	9	33.5	0.9
2 cups	410	14.7	758.9	58.5	12.8	0.6
2 cups	550	23.2	**1772**	69	25	1
5½ oz	488	44	259	76	79	3.2
7 oz	259	15	767	26.6	40	1
1 5-oz enchilada	426	24.5	**1084**	38.5	12.5	0.4
1 4½-oz enchilada	336.5	25	435	16.8	40	0.5
1 6-oz enchilada	496	31	784	38	60	1.2
1 oz	163.9	11.6	88.8	8.7	7.5	0.7
2 cups	100	4.5	269.5	32	0	2.7
10 oz	**791**	**44**	**842**	55	327	4.2
1 5-oz tostada	198.3	4.8	418.7	30.8	10	5

MEXICAN DISHES

FOOD NAME

Side Dishes
Lowest Fat: Colache—5 g fat, 88 calories
Highest Fat: Oaxacan Baked Black Beans—14 g fat, 555 calories

BANANA FRITTERS *Churros de Plátano*

CARROTS BAKED IN MILK *Zanahorias en Leche* with butter and parsley

COLACHE fresh corn cooked with zucchini, pepper, and tomatoes

FRIED BANANAS *Plátanos Fritos* with butter

GREEN BEANS WITH LEMON *Judías con Limón* with butter and parsley

LENTILS WITH PINEAPPLE AND BANANAS *Lentejas con Ananás y Plátanos* with chicken broth, celery, carrots, garlic, tomatoes, and raisins

OAXACAN BAKED BLACK BEANS *Frijoles Negros a la Oaxaca* with black beans, garlic, onion, cumin and ham hocks

STUFFED ZUCCHINI *Calabazas Rellenos* zucchini with cream cheese and sour cream

TOMATO RICE *Arroz de Tomate* with tomatoes, rice, peas and chorizo sausage

WHITE RICE *Arroz Blanco* toasted rice pilaf with oil, garlic, onion, and chicken stock

Beverages
Lowest Fat: Orange Sangría—0 g fat, 118 calories
Highest Fat: Mexican Hot Chocolate—23.2 g fat, 339 calories

CHI-CHI with rum, pineapple juice, and blackberry brandy

DAIQUIRI, BANANA with lime juice, sugar, rum, fresh fruit, banana liqueur, cream

Serving Size	Calories	Fat (g)	Sodium (mg)	Carbohydrate (g)	Cholesterol (mg)	Fiber (g)
½ banana	214	9	380	17.3	182.7	0.3
3 oz	99	5	752	11.2	15.8	0.7
6 oz	88	5	381	11.8	10.3	0.9
1 medium banana	138	6	59	22	15.5	0.5
4 oz	69	6	397	4.5	15.5	0.6
1½ cups	297	7	618.4	34	4.8	2
12 oz	555	14	**2019**	66.2	64.8	0.1
1 3-oz zucchini	174	13	398	11.4	15.5	1.3
1¼ cups	360	13.6	700	49.8	12.4	1.2
1½ cups	208	7	446	30.9	.3	0.2
7 oz	238.4	0.1	1.3	24.5	0	0.2
1 cup	289.1	4.8	6.4	23.2	16.6	0.1

MEXICAN DISHES

FOOD NAME

DAIQUIRI, BASIC FROZEN with lime juice, sugar, and rum

DAIQUIRI, STRAWBERRY with lime juice, sugar, rum, fresh strawberries, honey, and cream

MARGARITA with tequila, Triple Sec, sour mix, Kosher salt, and lime juice

MELÓN COLADA with rum, melon liqueur, coconut milk, pineapple juice, and cream

MEXICAN COFFEE with tequila and Kahlúa

MEXICAN HOT CHOCOLATE *Chocolate* with unsweetened chocolate, sugar, and cinnamon

PIÑA COLADA with coconut milk, pineapple juice, rum, and cream

SANGRÍA with red wine, club soda, assorted fruit, and sugar

SANGRÍA, ORANGE *Sangría de Naranja* with red wine, sugar, Cointreau, and oranges

TROPICAL FRUIT PUNCH *Ponche Tropical* with pineapple, orange, papaya, and guava

Desserts
Lowest Fat: Orange Candy—1 g fat, 50 calories
Highest Fat: Mexican Christmas Bread Pudding—26 g fat, 509 calories

BAKED PINEAPPLE WITH CUSTARD *Piña al Horno con Natillas* with sugar, rum, and butter, topped with chilled custard sauce

FLAN caramel custard with eggs, milk, sugar, and vanilla

CHEESE PUDDING IN CARAMEL SYRUP *Chongos Zamoranos* with milk, sugar, vanilla, rennet, and cinnamon

CHRISTMAS BREAD PUDDING *Pudín con Pan de Navidad* made with panettone, dried fruit, and Grand Marnier

Serving Size	Calories	Fat (g)	Sodium (mg)	Carbohydrate (g)	Cholesterol (mg)	Fiber (g)
1 cup	138.8	0	3	9	0	0
1 cup	359.7	5.2	8.1	40.2	16.6	0.8
5 oz	402	0	**1002**	19.8	0	0
9½ oz	337.8	11.2	24.9	22.2	16.6	0.1
1 cup	141.5	5.8	12.5	6.9	20	0
1 cup	**339**	**23.2**	173.3	33.2	33	0.3
9½ oz	273.7	11.4	24.4	16.9	18.8	0.3
4 oz	106.2	0.1	9.8	8.7	0.8	0.1
4 oz	118	0	7	14.9	0	0.1
1½ cups	222.4	0.7	16.5	40.9	2.3	3.8
8 oz	231	15	219	19.4	142.3	0.2
½ cup	213.3	8	109	26.2	285	0
1½ cups	500	13	192	84.8	52.8	0
5½ oz	**509**	**26**	339	59.6	167.1	0.5

MEXICAN DISHES

FOOD NAME

COCONUT FONDANT CANDY *Dulces de Coco* coconut with water and sugar, often tinted green or pink

COCONUT RICE PUDDING *Pudín de Coco y Arroz* with raisins and orange peel

CORN PUDDING *Pudín de Elote* with eggs, sugar, cinnamon, and vanilla

EMPANADA, PUMPKIN-RAISIN *Empanada de Calabaza y Pasa* pastry with flour, shortening, sugar, and anise, stuffed with pumpkin, raisins, and sugar

EMPANADA, CHEESE-CURRANT *Empanada de Queso y Pasa de Corinto* as above, with cottage cheese and golden raisins

MANGO CREAM *Crema de Mango* with oranges, heavy cream, and pecans

ORANGE CANDY *Dulces de Naranja* made with evaporated milk, orange peel, and walnuts

PRICKLY PEAR DESSERT *Postre de Tunas* sliced and served with lime juice and whipped cream

Basics
Lowest Fat: Salsa Carnaval—0 g fat, 6 calories
Highest Fat: Refried Beans with Cheese—60 g fat, 633 calories

CHILE-TOMATO SAUCE with onion, oil, tomato puree, garlic, chile, cumin, and oregano

CILANTRO MAYONNAISE with sour cream, orange zest, parsley, salt, and pepper

GUACAMOLE with avocado, lemon, salt, cilantro, and chilies

MOLE SAUCE chili powder and chocolate

NUT SAUCE *Nogada* with walnuts, heavy cream, almonds, parsley, cinnamon, and salt

Serving Size	Calories	Fat (g)	Sodium (mg)	Carbohydrate (g)	Cholesterol (mg)	Fiber (g)
4 candies	132	2	4	29.2	0	0.2
¾ cup	361	8	135	60.8	21	0.3
½ cup	184	5	183	31.5	205.5	0.3
1 1½-oz empanada	209	12	253	19.5	0	0.3
1 2½-oz empanada	237	13	328	23.4	25.4	0.2
½ cup	283	21	17	23.6	54.3	1.05
1 1-inch piece	50	1	14	9.6	1.2	.03
pulp from 1 prickly pear	337	23	34	33.7	81.5	3.7
2 tblsp	44.3	1.4	181.5	7.7	0	0.3
2 tblsp	131.4	14	153.6	1.4	6.4	0
2 tblsp	98.8	9.3	308.8	4.8	0	1.3
2 tblsp	60.5	5.3	228.8	2.9	7.8	0
2 tblsp	87.3	8.3	164.1	2	13.7	0.1

MEXICAN DISHES

FOOD NAME
RED CHILE SAUCE *Salsa de Chile Rojo* with tomato paste, garlic, and oil
REFRIED BEANS *Frijoles Refritos* pinto beans and onions fried in butter
REFRIED BEANS FRIED IN VEGETABLE OIL
REFRIED BEANS WITH CHEESE fried in butter, with Cheddar cheese
SALSA *Salsa Cruda* with tomatoes and green chilies
SALSA CARNAVAL with cantaloupe, watermelon, cucumber, and tomatoes
SALSA, CORN *Salsa de Elote* with papaya, onion, and tomatoes
SALSA, GREEN TOMATILLO *Salsa de Tomatillo* with onions, almonds, oil, cilantro, and chicken broth
SOUR CREAM
TORTILLAS, CORN *Tortillas de Maíz* fried crisp
TORTILLAS, CORN baked
TORTILLAS, FLOUR *Tortillas de Harina* baked, with salt and lard
TORTILLAS, FLOUR fried crisp

Serving Size	Calories	Fat (g)	Sodium (mg)	Carbohydrate (g)	Cholesterol (mg)	Fiber (g)
2 tblsp	21.6	2	176.8	1	0	0.1
1 cup	356	16	496	40.3	41.3	2.7
1 cup	390	19	7	40.3	0	2.7
1 cup	**633**	**60**	786	36.6	143.7	2.3
2 tblsp	9.1	0	169.6	2	0	0.1
2 tblsp	6	0	1.2	1.4	0	0.1
2 tblsp	9.8	0.1	1.5	2.3	0	0.1
2 tblsp	35.6	2.5	80.4	2.5	0.1	0.3
2 tblsp	61.6	6	15.4	2.5	12.8	0
1 6-inch tortilla	123	7.4	0	13.5	0	0.3
1 6-inch tortilla	63	0.6	0	13.5	0	0.3
1 7-inch tortilla	148.5	6.3	199.8	12	5.5	0.1
1 7-inch tortilla	218.5	15.3	0	13.5	0	0.3

Russian and Eastern European Cuisine

Like German food, Russian and Eastern European cuisine tends to be heavy, and delicious. The trick in these restaurants is to order selectively. Borscht, a popular beet soup served in many Polish, Ukranian and Russian restaurants, is always a good choice for a starter. A cup has 2.7 grams of fat, and this soup will fill you up so that you eat less of the more caloric entrees that follow. Ask for your borscht to be served without the dollop of sour cream in the center.

Since the Russian Orthodox Church has up to 250 religious days a year when eating meat is not allowed, fish and vegetable dishes have become staples in the Russian diet—a special bonus for diners looking for low-fat meals. Smoked fish is popular and healthy, and root vegetable dishes which include either potatoes, cabbage, carrots, turnips or a combination of several of these, abound throughout Eastern Europe. Even if you've never been impressed by cabbage, you should try some of these wonderful dishes. Smoking and boiling are both popular cooking methods in Russia and Eastern Europe, and dishes prepared this way are usually low in fat.

RUSSIAN AND EASTERN EUROPEAN DISHES

FOOD NAME

Soups
Lowest Fat: *Beet Soup—2.7 g fat, 69.8 calories*
Highest Fat: *Sauerkraut Soup—8.4 g fat, 102.4 calories*

BEET SOUP *Borscht* with beets, carrots, onions, butter, beef stock, cabbage, and vinegar

CABBAGE SOUP with cabbage, onion, butter, beef broth, and grated Cheddar

MATZO BALL CHICKEN SOUP with chicken, carrots, onions, celery, parsley, dill, eggs, and matzo meal

SAUERKRAUT SOUP with cabbage, onion, butter, beef broth, tomatoes, and sour cream

Main Dishes
Lowest Fat: *Black Beef Brisket—14.6 g fat, 285.1 calories*
Highest Fat: *Chicken Kiev—74.6 g fat, 981.4 calories*

BLACK BEEF BRISKET with beef, onions, carrots, bay leaf, cayenne, cumin, and white peppercorns

CABBAGE ROLLS WITH LEMON SAUCE stuffed with cabbage, onion, butter, ground beef, rice, lemon juice, and flour

CHICKEN KIEV chicken breasts deep-fried with butter, chives, parsley, garlic, flour, egg, and bread crumbs

CHICKEN PAPRIKASH chicken simmered with butter, oil, onions, paprika, chicken broth, flour, and sour cream

GOULASH, BEEF with beef, butter, onions, green pepper, and paprika

GOULASH, HUNGARIAN with beef chuck, onion, green pepper, butter, paprika, cider vinegar, and beef stock

GOULASH, LAMB with lamb, butter, onions, caraway, marjoram, garlic, and paprika

Serving Size	Calories	Fat (g)	Sodium (mg)	Carbohydrate (g)	Cholesterol (mg)	Fiber (g)
1 cup	69.8	2.7	382.4	9.7	6.2	0.8
1 cup	93.8	8.1	743.5	2.2	22.1	0.2
1 cup	154.6	7.9	112.1	12.7	95.9	1.4
1 cup	102.4	**8.4**	**1184.4**	6.5	19.5	0.9
6 oz	285.1	14.6	159.1	2.5	98	0.1
3 2½-oz rolls	573.9	41.9	**1969.3**	25.1	117	0.4
8 oz	**981.4**	**74.6**	964.5	8.6	**376.5**	0.1
8 oz	790.1	52.7	**1157.7**	12.2	246.2	0.3
1 cup	393.1	24.2	631.4	5	113	0.3
1 cup	533.2	42.8	**1081.7**	3.3	139.9	0.3
1 cup	517.5	46.2	356.6	4.3	131.3	0.3

RUSSIAN AND EASTERN EUROPEAN DISHES

FOOD NAME

GOULASH, PORK AND VEAL, WITH SAUERKRAUT with pork, veal, cabbage, onions, butter, caraway seeds, and sour cream

PIROGIES Flour, egg, and sour cream dumplings with onion, butter, mushrooms, and ground beef

PIROZHKI with puff pastry, egg yolk, onions, olive oil, beef chuck, beef broth, sour cream, flour, dill and parsley

PORK CHOPS PAPRIKA WITH SOUR CREAM GRAVY with onion, beef broth, and bay leaf

ROAST LOIN OF PORK WITH PARSNIP-SOUR CREAM SAUCE roast pork with celery, parsnip, onion, white wine, butter, and flour

STEAK ESTERHÁZY beef with flour, butter, carrot, mushrooms, celery, onion, parsley, capers, and sour cream

VEAL AND CHESTNUT STEW with veal, chestnut, butter, onion, garlic, chicken broth, white wine, and thyme

Side Dishes
Lowest Fat: *Kosher Dill Pickles—0.1 g fat, 16 calories*
Highest Fat: *Potato Pancakes—23.6 g fat, 251.6 calories*

BOILED BEETS IN SOUR CREAM beets with horseradish, chives and onion

BUCKWHEAT GROATS *Kasha* with butter

GEFILTE FISH with whitefish, onion, celery, carrots, parsley, eggs, and matzo meal

KIELBASA Polish pork sausage with garlic

KOSHER DILL PICKLES cucumbers with white vinegar, pickling salt, garlic, and dill seed

LEEK PANCAKES with ground beef, leek, bread crumbs, parsley and cumin

Serving Size	Calories	Fat (g)	Sodium (mg)	Carbohydrate (g)	Cholesterol (mg)	Fiber (g)
1 cup	286.7	23.9	364.6	3.9	75.9	0.5
9 oz	**846.9**	**67.5**	**999.7**	38.1	165.3	1.4
3 pirozhki	195.0	8.6	192.9	12.8	56.4	.13
1 4-oz chop	527.5	46.6	220.5	3.9	122	0.1
8 oz	**976.1**	**69.5**	**980.2**	7.3	253.3	0.4
8 oz	**895.9**	**59.9**	**1817.2**	20.4	236	0.7
1½ cups	688.3	28.9	**1085.8**	52.6	162.9	1.4
½ cup	72.3	4.1	130.3	7.7	8.5	0.5
¾ cup	192.3	6.9	63	30.7	15.5	0.8
2 2-oz balls	117	5.2	162.3	2.2	95.6	0.1
1 oz	88	7.7	305	0.6	19	0
5 oz	16	0.1	400.5	2.9	0	0.4
4 1-oz pancakes	251.6	18.4	430.4	7.2	109.6	0.7

RUSSIAN AND EASTERN EUROPEAN DISHES

FOOD NAME

POTATO PANCAKES *Latkes* with potatoes, onion, eggs, and flour and fried in corn oil

RUSSIAN RAISED PANCAKES *Blini* with milk, sugar, flour, egg, and butter

SALMON AND KASHA *Coulibiac* with salmon, kasha, scallions, mushrooms, hard-boiled eggs, butter, flour, tomato puree, chervil, tarragon, and parsley

Desserts
Lowest Fat: Blintzes with Cottage Cheese—7.8 g fat, 175.8 calories
Highest Fat: Vanilla Cream Charlotte—48.8 g fat, 546.1 calories

ALMOND KISSEL *Kisel iz Mindalya* pudding with sweet and bitter almonds, sugar, and potato flour

BLINTZES WITH COTTAGE CHEESE Pancakes with flour, sugar, milk, eggs, butter, vanilla, sugar, and cinnamon

DRUM TORTE *Doboš* with butter, eggs, sugar, flour, vanilla and chocolate

RUGELACH cream-cheese cookies with butter, sugar, flour, egg, vanilla, and lemon juice

VANILLA CREAM CHARLOTTE *Vanil'nyi Krem Sharlot* with milk, sugar, egg, butter and brandy

Serving Size	Calories	Fat (g)	Sodium (mg)	Carbohydrate (g)	Cholesterol (mg)	Fiber (g)
4 1-oz pancakes	**251.6**	**23.6**	306.8	33.8	188.2	1.7
2 2-inch pancakes	244.2	13.9	715.3	13.3	273.1	0.1
5 oz	275	14.1	805	21.9	108.8	0.2
1 cup	**498.1**	**28.9**	2.3	56.8	0	1.4
2 5-inch cakes	175.8	7.8	495.4	12.9	119.4	0.1
1 2-inch slice	384.8	27.1	233.3	28.9	274.8	0.1
5 small cookies	426.4	27.4	126	32.5	101.8	0.1
½ cup	**546.1**	**48.8**	55.4	25.9	198	0

Spanish Cuisine

Many Spanish restaurants offer *tapas*—little plates of bite-sized appetizers that are often eaten in place of a meal. Many of these items are low in fat and can provide calorie-conscious eaters with the opportunity to sample lots of goodies in small portions. *Paella* is also a popular Spanish staple and is prepared hundreds of different ways—the only constants are saffron and rice. These two ingredients are served in a casserole as a main course with seafood, vegetables, chorizo sausage, pork, beef, or game—or all of these. Of course, the fat and calorie counts of the many paella presentations vary widely depending on what the individual dish contains, so be sure to ask your server what the chef includes in his version. Spanish dishes can be very complicated, requiring twenty or more ingredients, and the result is a flavorful and unique cuisine that features many healthy fish and vegetable dishes. Look for foods that are roasted, broiled, grilled, or stewed and try to steer clear of some of the pastas, which, atypically for Spanish cuisine, are loaded with cheese.

SPANISH DISHES

FOOD NAME

Appetizers (Tapas)
Lowest Fat: Scallop Cocktail with Lime—1 g fat, 105 calories
Highest Fat: Marinated Fish—21 g fat, 303 calories

BREAD WITH TOMATOES (FROM CATALUÑA) *Pa amb Tomaquet* with crusty bread, tomatoes, garlic, and olive oil

SHRIMP APPETIZER *Aperitivo de Camaron* deep-fried shrimp, in egg-and-bread-crumb batter

HAM FRITTERS *Buñuelitos* with ham, pimiento, onion, bread crumbs, eggs, and flour, and deep-fried

MARINATED FISH *Escabeche* fish with chilies, garlic, vinegar, and orange juice

MEAT-FILLED TURNOVERS *Empanaditas* with ground veal, onion, ham, pimiento, olives, and red hot liquid seasoning, deep-fried

ORANGE AND ONION SALAD *Ensalada de Naranjas* seasoned with chili powder

SCALLOP COCKTAIL WITH LIME *Mariscos con Lima* scallops with white wine, lime juice, catsup, and cayenne

Vegetable Dishes
Lowest Fat: Sautéed Green Peppers—4 g fat, 58 calories
Highest Fat: Baked Asparagus—25.5 g fat, 278.7 calories

ASPARAGUS, BAKED with asparagus, eggs, pimientos, lemon juice, light cream, and chives

BROCCOLI, SAUTÉED WITH RIPE OLIVES with broccoli, olives, garlic, olive oil, and butter

EGGPLANT, PEPPERS, AND TOMATOES, BASQUE-STYLE with eggplant, peppers, tomatoes, olive oil, salt, and parsley

GREEN PEPPERS, SAUTÉED green peppers fried in butter

Serving Size	Calories	Fat (g)	Sodium (mg)	Carbohydrate (g)	Cholesterol (mg)	Fiber (g)
2 slices	224.5	8.6	404.6	32.2	0	0.4
1 jumbo or 2 medium shrimp	94	7	235	2	76	0
2 ½-oz fritters	67.1	4.9	268.1	1.8	42.6	.02
5 oz	**303**	**21**	560	3.8	65.3	0.1
2 turnovers, ½-oz each	142.7	12.0	206.9	5.5	9.0	.09
½ cup	135	9	251	14	0	0.5
5 oz	105	1	428	5.6	32	0.1
8 6-oz spears	**278.7**	**25.5**	190	7.4	194.9	1.1
1 cup	137.9	12.6	402.8	6.4	7.8	1.7
1 cup	126.6	9.5	367.2	9.4	0	1.1
1 7-oz green pepper	58	4	43	6	10	1.2

SPANISH DISHES

FOOD NAME

RICE, SPANISH-STYLE rice with onions, sweet green peppers, chili powder, tomatoes, and bay leaf

Soups and Stews
Lowest Fat: Basque Cabbage Soup—5.7 g fat, 89.2 calories
Highest Fat: Tomato-Pepper Cream Soup—20 g fat, 281.6 calories

BASQUE CABBAGE SOUP with cabbage, onions, beef broth, lima beans, garlic, and vinegar

CLEAR GAZPACHO with chicken broth, tomatoes, onion, pepper, and celery

PORK AND VEGETABLE SOUP *Garbure* with salt pork, garlic, celery, parsley, carrots, potatoes, lima beans, white kidney beans, and cabbage

TOMATO-PEPPER CREAM SOUP *Caldo Largo* with tomato, peppers, chicken broth, evaporated milk, and Monterey Jack cheese

VEGETABLE STEW *Pisto* with ham, olive oil, onions, sweet red peppers, pimientos, eggplant, mushrooms, artichoke hearts, and tomatoes

Main Dishes
Lowest Fat: Chicken with Rice—25.2 g fat, 455.9 calories
Highest Fat: Green-Mole—65 g fat, 883 calories

BEEF CATALAN beef with onions, carrots, turnips, cinnamon, cloves, tomatoes, red wine, cannellini beans, and parsley

CHICKEN MOLE *Mole de Pollo* chicken with onions, garlic, chicken broth, chili powder, almonds, banana, cinnamon, sesame seeds, unsweetened chocolate, and pine nuts

CHICKEN WITH ORANGES, RAISINS, AND ALMONDS *Pollo con Naranjas* chicken baked, with onions, orange juice, saffron, capers, cinnamon, and cloves

CHICKEN WITH RICE *Arroz con Pollo* with chicken, rice, tomatoes, peas, asparagus, salt pork, onion, butter, garlic, and olive oil

Serving Size	Calories	Fat (g)	Sodium (mg)	Carbohydrate (g)	Cholesterol (mg)	Fiber (g)
1¼ cups	196.7	7.3	541.3	28.2	0	0.9
1 cup	89.2	5.7	871.8	5.9	13.8	0.5
1 cup	118.4	7.2	**1046.4**	10.2	0.8	1
1 cup	**369.5**	16.7	**852.2**	41.1	42.1	2.39
1 cup	281.6	**20**	543.2	35.5	26.2	0.7
1 cup	131.8	8.2	468.7	12.1	4.9	1
2 cups	**888.0**	49.4	**1044.7**	29.6	158.8	2.22
2 cups	507	36	**1005**	14	122	0.6
10 oz	472	29.3	241	12	117	0.6
8 oz	455.9	25.2	729.6	31.6	79.4	0.5

SPANISH DISHES

FOOD NAME

GREEN MOLE *Mole Verde* pork with tomatillo sauce, lettuce, pickled chilies, and sour cream

PAELLA WITH PORK, SAUSAGE, AND SEAFOOD rice with clams, shrimp, pork, sausage, lime, butter, garlic, and spices

PAELLA WITH CHICKEN with rice, chicken, olive oil, onions, saffron, garlic, red peppers, chorizo, shrimp, and clams

PAELLA WITH SEAFOOD with rice, olive oil, onions, saffron, tomatoes, garlic, parsley, clams, mussels, squid, shrimp, and fish stock

SWORDFISH *Pescado España al Horno a la Manzanillo* swordfish with olive oil and sliced green onions

Desserts
Lowest Fat: Pastry Puffs—10 g fat, 307 calories
Highest Fat: Almond Pudding with Custard Sauce—19 g fat, 362 calories

ALMOND PUDDING WITH CUSTARD SAUCE *Almendrado* with eggs, milk, sugar, and lemon peel

BREAD PUDDING *Capirotada* with bread, raisins, walnuts, and Cheddar cheese

MILK PUDDING *Leche Quemada* with vanilla or almond extract

PASTRY PUFFS *Buñuelos* fried pastry made with flour, sugar, butter, eggs, and milk

Serving Size	Calories	Fat (g)	Sodium (mg)	Carbohydrate (g)	Cholesterol (mg)	Fiber (g)
11 oz	**883**	**65**	487	33	164.5	1.3
2 cups	**808**	41	**2122**	64	164	1.3
1½ cups	446.9	16.2	694.3	43	100.3	0.3
1½ cups	747	26.2	**1023.3**	52.5	**521.5**	0.9
1 8-oz steak	468	29.5	**1707**	4.5	87.5	0.4
5 oz	362	**19**	99	40.2	239.3	0.6
1 cup	361	16	203	35.9	23.4	0.4
½ cup	**690**	10.7	160	142	44	0
2 oz (4 small puffs)	307	10	584	47.6	86.1	0.1

Thai Cuisine

Like other Southeast Asian cuisines, Thai cooking relies heavily on rice and noodles for bulk. In addition to rice, the coconut is one of Thailand's principal agricultural products and plays a significant role in the country's cuisine. Both the meat and the milk of coconuts are high in fat; and, along with fried foods, they should be avoided or eaten only occasionally and in very small portions. The good news is that there are usually plenty of low-fat alternatives on Thai menus that you can enjoy without sacrificing variety and taste. For example, while the typical Thai spring roll is stuffed with a minced-meat mixture and deep-fried, there are also larger rolls—sometimes called Thai salad rolls—that are wrapped in rice paper and served cold. These tasty low-fat treats contain vermicelli (also called glass noodles), vegetables, and often a shrimp or two. If you are in the mood for meat, consider fish instead: a 4-ounce delicious red snapper fillet provides a comparatively low 12 grams of fat, as opposed to the 34 grams found in the same amount of Thai beef salad. Ask for steamed rather than fried vegetables. Steaming locks in nutrients and allows you to avoid additional oil. For dessert, stick to fresh fruit. Fresh mango slices, served in many Thai restaurants, have about 40 times less fat than mango ice cream, and they are just as sweet.

THAI DISHES

FOOD NAME

Appetizers
Lowest Fat: *Scallops with Lime—4.6 g fat, 128 calories*
Highest Fat: *Corn Cakes—51.6 g fat, 565.3 calories*

BEEF SATAY skewered beef with peanut sauce

CHICKEN SATAY skewered chicken with peanut sauce

CORN CAKES with corn, green curry paste, green onions, and fish sauce, deep fried in vegetable oil

CRAB ROLLS with chicken, crabmeat, green onions, bean sprouts, carrot, and fish sauce, wrapped in rice paper and deep-fried

FRIED DUMPLING wonton skins filled with shrimp, water chestnuts, green onions, and fish sauce, deep fried in vegetable oil

PORK SATAY with pork, lime juice, lemon grass, garlic, peanuts, shallots, fish paste, and coconut milk

SCALLOPS WITH LIME scallops with garlic, shallots, red chili, palm sugar, and fish sauce

THAI SPRING ROLL deep-fried and stuffed with minced pork, bean sprouts, and vermicelli

Soups
Lowest Fat: *Vermicelli Soup—1.6 g fat, 106.5 calories*
Highest Fat: *Chicken and Coconut Soup—73.4 g fat, 804.2 calories*

CHICKEN AND COCONUT SOUP *Tohm Kah Gai* with boneless skinless chicken, coconut milk, lemon grass, green onions, red chilies, lime juice, fish sauce, and cilantro

LEMON GRASS SOUP *Tohm Yum* with shrimp, fish stock, lime juice, fish sauce, and red and green chilies

PORK AND PEANUT SOUP with lean chopped pork, cilantro, garlic, green onions, veal stock, raw peanuts, Chinese black mushrooms, bamboo shoots, and fish sauce

Serving Size	Calories	Fat (g)	Sodium (mg)	Carbohydrate (g)	Cholesterol (mg)	Fiber (g)
6 oz	227.9	14.8	81.8	0.3	59.5	0
6 oz	195.3	14.7	86.9	0.3	97.3	.05
2 cakes	565.3	51.6	203.2	24.0	60.9	.68
2 rolls	438.1	40.3	306.2	6.5	40.4	.16
3 dumplings	541.4	49.0	131.9	19.5	38.5	.17
3 oz	474.5	36.6	136.8	11.8	76	0.59
4 scallops in shells	128.0	4.6	239.6	4.6	32.0	.09
1 small roll	83.8	5.7	84.4	5.1	21.9	0.25
1 cup	319	26	308.2	13.2	24.5	0.05
1 cup	103.3	4.0	775.1	3.1	76.4	0
1¼ cups	304.0	**22.0**	**964.2**	5.3	57.9	1.23

THAI DISHES

FOOD NAME

THAI CHICKEN AND MUSHROOM SOUP with chicken pieces, garlic, cilantro, chicken stock, Chinese black mushrooms, fish sauce, and green onions

VERMICELLI SOUP *Gaeng Jued Woon Sen* with chicken stock, onion, lemon grass, lime juice, garlic, chilies, fish sauce, vermicelli, and cilantro

Salads
Lowest Fat: Hot Bamboo-Shoot Salad—0.3 g fat, 30.2 calories
Highest Fat: Pork and Bamboo-Shoot Salad—26 g fat, 337.4 calories

BEAN SALAD with lime juice, fish sauce, nam prik, peanuts, garlic, red chili, and coconut cream

CHICKEN AND MINT SALAD with chicken, lemon grass, chilies, lime juice, fish sauce, and palm sugar

HOT BAMBOO-SHOOT SALAD with bamboo shoots, fish sauce, palm sugar, garlic, and rice

PORK AND BAMBOO-SHOOT SALAD with pork, bamboo shoots, garlic, onion, egg, fish sauce, palm sugar, and lime juice

SHRIMP SALAD WITH MINT with shrimp, lime, palm sugar, fish sauce, red curry paste, lemon grass, coconut cream, mint, and cucumber

SQUID SALAD *Yum Pla Merk* with bell pepper, chilies, fish sauce, lime juice, palm sugar, garlic, lemon grass, mint, and cilantro

THAI BEEF SALAD with beef, rice, fish sauce, lime juice, palm sugar, green chilies, and garlic

Serving Size	Calories	Fat (g)	Sodium (mg)	Carbohydrate (g)	Cholesterol (mg)	Fiber (g)
1¼ cups	134.2	7.9	**1112.7**	2.3	25.6	.23
1½ cups	106.5	1.6	**1066.4**	15.8	1.0	.09
½ cup	155.7	12.4	543.4	8.0	18.6	.70
½ cup	243.4	9.3	303.7	2.6	97.3	.09
½ cup	30.2	0.3	349.1	6.2	0.0	1.30
½ cup	**337.4**	26.0	317.2	7.2	136.2	1.40
5 shrimp	**416.1**	9.4	546.0	47.9	260.0	.34
¾ cup	312.6	17.6	645.3	14.4	336.6	.34
½ cup	277.5	19.4	306.7	6.9	66.6	.21

THAI DISHES

FOOD NAME

Noodles and Rice

Lowest Fat: Rice, Chicken, and Mushrooms—9.2 g fat, 266.1 calories
Highest Fat: Crispy Noodles—37.6 g fat, 569.3 calories

CRISPY NOODLES *Mee-Grob* made with rice vermicelli, Chinese black mushrooms, pork, chicken breast, eggs, garlic, bean sprouts, lime juice, and fish sauce

NOODLES, CRAB, AND EGGPLANT with egg-thread noodles, garlic, green chili, fish sauce, lime juice, and cilantro

NOODLES, PORK, AND SHRIMP with bean-thread noodles, Chinese black mushrooms, shallots, celery, fish sauce, lime juice, palm sugar, red chilies, and cilantro

NOODLES, PORK, AND BROCCOLI with rice noodles, garlic, peanuts, and fish sauce

NOODLES WITH HERB SAUCE with egg noodles, peanuts, green chili, garlic, basil, mint, cilantro, lime juice, and fish sauce

RICE, CHICKEN, AND MUSHROOMS with rice, onion, garlic, red chilies, bamboo shoots, dried shrimp, fish sauce, and basil leaves

RICE, SHRIMP, AND BEAN CURD with garlic, onion, red chilies, fish sauce, and shallots

SPICY FRIED RICE with onion, garlic, green chilies, red curry paste, pork, shrimp, eggs, and fish sauce

THAI FRIED NOODLES *Nam Prik* with rice vermicelli, garlic, fish sauce, lime juice, eggs, shrimp, bean sprouts, and peanuts

THAI FRIED RICE *Kao Pahd* with rice, green beans, onions, garlic, pork, chicken, eggs, nam prik, fish sauce, shrimp, and cilantro

Serving Size	Calories	Fat (g)	Sodium (mg)	Carbohydrate (g)	Cholesterol (mg)	Fiber (g)
8 oz	**569.3**	**37.6**	313.5	33.0	202.8	.99
8 oz	250.3	14.7	694.1	30.8	60.9	.57
9 oz	427.8	24.9	601.0	14.6	178.9	.81
9 oz	332.0	22.8	190.6	13.7	63.2	.56
8 oz	359.0	30.5	74.2	18.7	21.9	.25
8 oz	266.1	9.2	271.0	22.9	59.4	.99
8 oz	255.4	12.3	381.3	23.4	65.0	.21
8 oz	286.6	14.3	347.5	23.8	250.7	.19
9 oz	516.2	23.5	320.8	54.5	201.7	.87
8 oz	374.4	18.7	578.6	25.9	228.4	.41

THAI DISHES

FOOD NAME

Vegetable Dishes
Lowest Fat: Mushrooms and Bean Sprouts—8 g fat, 117.6 calories
Highest Fat: Spiced Cabbage—27.2 g fat, 316.5 calories

BROCCOLI WITH SHRIMP *Pahd Ka-Nah* with shrimp, broccoli, peanut oil, garlic, red chili, and fish sauce

CUCUMBER SALAD with cucumber, peanuts, red chili, green chili, shallot, dried shrimp, and lime juice and peel

MUSHROOMS AND BEAN SPROUTS with mushrooms, bean sprouts, red chilies, garlic, shrimp, lime juice, shallots, fish sauce, rice, cilantro, and mint

SPICED CABBAGE with cabbage, coconut cream, shallots, pork, coconut milk, fish sauce, and red chili

STIR-FRIED SNOW PEAS with snow peas, garlic, pork, palm sugar, fish sauce, and shrimp

STUFFED EGGPLANT with eggplant, garlic, lemon grass, onion, chicken breasts, fish sauce, and basil

STUFFED ZUCCHINI with zucchini, coconut, cilantro, chili, vegetable oil, lime juice, and fish sauce

TOSSED SPINACH with peanut oil, chicken, garlic, fish sauce, and peanuts

VEGETABLES WITH SAUCE *Pahd Puk* with eggplant, green beans, cauliflower, coconut milk, coconut cream, peanuts, and fish sauce

Egg Dishes
Lowest Fat: Stuffed Eggs—8.6 g fat, 137.3 calories
Highest Fat: Son-in-Law Eggs—23.7 g fat, 248.3 calories

EGG NESTS with eggs, cilantro, garlic, peanut oil, onions, pork, shrimp, fish sauce, and chilies

SON-IN-LAW EGGS hard-cooked eggs, onion, fish sauce, sugar, and red chili

Serving Size	Calories	Fat (g)	Sodium (mg)	Carbohydrate (g)	Cholesterol (mg)	Fiber (g)
5 oz	137.5	10.8	270.3	4.1	43.2	.48
4 oz	161.8	11.2	237.7	4.6	74.3	.37
5 oz	117.6	8.0	260.6	5.0	43.2	.83
8 oz	316.5	27.2	231.9	12.3	22.5	5.88
5 oz	193.6	12.7	259.8	7.1	46.7	2.24
½ eggplant	150.5	8.5	179.2	4.5	36.5	.49
8 oz	267.8	17.7	27.3	28.4	0.0	3.08
8 oz	200.7	14.2	393.2	3.3	49.0	.28
9 oz	146.7	12.2	168.6	9.3	0.0	0.43
4 oz	271.8	22.3	240.1	1.4	205.7	.04
1 egg	248.3	23.7	357.4	2.9	274.0	.04

THAI DISHES

FOOD NAME

STEAMED EGGS   with eggs, green onions, shrimp, chili, cilantro, coconut milk, and fish sauce
STUFFED EGGS   with eggs, pork, shrimp, fish sauce, garlic, and cilantro
STUFFED OMELET   with eggs, onions, garlic, cilantro, pork, green beans, and fish sauce

Chicken Dishes
Lowest Fat: Barbecued Chicken—10.7 g fat, 279.7 calories
Highest Fat: Stuffed Chicken Wings—66.7 g fat, 741.9 calories

BARBECUED CHICKEN   *Gai Yang*   with chicken, red chilies, garlic, shallots, palm sugar, coconut cream, and fish sauce
CHICKEN AND WATERCRESS   *Pra Ram Rong Sohng*   with garlic, fish sauce, lime juice, palm sugar, peanut oil, dried shrimp, and roasted peanuts
CHICKEN IN COCONUT MILK   chicken with cilantro, green chilies, coconut milk, lime, and fish sauce
CHICKEN IN PEANUT SAUCE   chicken with garlic, curry paste, coconut cream, shallots, roast peanuts, coconut milk, and fish sauce
CHICKEN WITH BASIL   chicken with garlic, onion, red chilies, fish sauce, coconut milk, and lime juice
CHICKEN WITH CILANTRO   chicken with garlic, lime, and fish sauce
CHICKEN WITH GALANGAL   with chicken, garlic, onion, Chinese black mushrooms, red chili, fish sauce, palm sugar, and lime juice
CHICKEN WITH LEMON GRASS   chicken with green onions, green chili, and fish sauce
CHICKEN WITH SNOW PEAS   with chicken, garlic, red chilies, shallots, lime juice, fish sauce, lemon grass, and brown rice

Serving Size	Calories	Fat (g)	Sodium (mg)	Carbohydrate (g)	Cholesterol (mg)	Fiber (g)
8 oz	184.7	10.9	333.8	6.3	408.7	0.56
one 3-oz egg	137.3	8.6	173.6	1.6	308.3	.10
8 oz (2 eggs)	264.1	19.9	246.4	3.4	463.7	.23
1 6-oz chicken breast	279.7	10.7	250.1	7.9	97.3	.28
1 cup	324.7	19.3	410.9	5.0	167.4	.29
10 oz	352.8	22.5	254.9	5.1	112	0
1¼ cups	497.8	32	278	13.6	97.3	.77
1¼ cups	364.1	18.6	453.8	4.1	116.8	0.13
2 pieces (9 oz)	241.3	12.7	353.0	2.0	118.0	.04
1 cup	299.7	14.5	303.2	4.5	97.3	.68
8 oz	400.5	23.7	263.8	0.9	156.8	.07
¾ cup	340.2	21.7	248.3	10.9	84.0	1.27

THAI DISHES

FOOD NAME

SPICED CHICKEN   with shallots, garlic, cilantro, lemon grass, red chilies, ginger, and shrimp paste

STUFFED CHICKEN WINGS   with chicken, pork, shrimp, green onions, garlic, cilantro, and fish sauce, deep-fried in vegetable oil

PORK DISHES
Lowest Fat: Vegetables and Pork—18.08 g fat, 256.5 calories
Highest Fat: Barbecued Spareribs— 49.9 g fat, 623.9 calories

BARBECUED SPARERIBS   with spareribs, cilantro, garlic, lime peel, green curry paste, fish sauce, palm sugar, and coconut milk

PORK AND BAMBOO SHOOTS   with pork, garlic, peanuts, fish sauce, and green onions

PORK AND BEAN STIR-FRY   with pork, garlic, water chestnuts, shrimp, and fish sauce

PORK AND NOODLE BALLS   with egg thread noodles, ground pork, garlic, cilantro, and fish sauce, deep-fried in vegetable oil

PORK TOASTS   with pork, shrimp, garlic, cilantro, green onions, eggs, fish sauce, brea, and coconut milk, deep fried in vegetable oil

PORK WITH GREEN ONIONS   with coconut milk, fish sauce, peanuts, red chilies, garlic, lemon grass, coconut cream, and spinach

PORK WITH WATER CHESTNUTS   with garlic, red chilies, fish sauce, cilantro, and green onions

VEGETABLES AND PORK   with pork, garlic, snow peas, broccoli, red bell pepper, zucchini and fish sauce

Serving Size	Calories	Fat (g)	Sodium (mg)	Carbohydrate (g)	Cholesterol (mg)	Fiber (g)
1 4-oz piece	250.1	17.8	111.2	4.0	78.9	.36
1 chicken wing	**741.9**	**66.7**	494.0	18.6	78.7	.21
6 ribs (8 oz)	**623.9**	**49.9**	233.3	9.2	129.6	0.05
⅔ cup	359.7	27.7	204.8	4.0	76.0	.86
1 cup	347.5	23.8	332.0	4.6	119.2	.56
3 balls	456.0	42.2	251.7	5.1	125.3	.06
3 oz	396.6	32.3	277.7	11.8	157.3	.52
1¼ cups	605.4	**46.2**	289.3	16.6	81.0	11.57
⅔ cup	336.6	24.6	163.2	2.8	86.9	.45
¾ cup	256.5	18.0	260.2	8.4	50.7	1.24

THAI DISHES

FOOD NAME

Curry Dishes
Lowest Fat: Shrimp and Cucumber Curry—17 g fat, 259.7 calories
Highest Fat: Duck Curry—105.9 g fat, 1106.5 calories

BEEF CURRY with beef, red curry paste, lemon grass, green beans, Chinese black mushrooms, peanuts, green chili, fish sauce, and palm sugar

DUCK CURRY with duck, coconut cream, green curry paste, coconut milk, fish sauce, green chili, and basil

LEMON-GRASS CHICKEN CURRY with chicken, lemon grass, red curry paste, garlic, fish sauce, and palm sugar

SHRIMP AND CUCUMBER CURRY with shrimp, cucumber, coconut cream, red curry paste, coconut milk, and palm sugar

STEAMED CHICKEN CURRY with chicken, curry paste, coconut milk, lime leaves, and basil leaves

THAI PORK CURRY with pork, coconut cream, onion, garlic, curry paste, fish sauce, palm sugar, basil, and lime leaves

Seafood
Lowest Fat: Shrimp with Mushrooms—2.6 g fat, 164.8 calories
Highest Fat: Fish with Mushroom Sauce—46.9 g fat, 914.7 calories

DEEP-FRIED COCONUT SHRIMP shrimp coated with rice flour, coconut, egg, coconut milk, and fish sauce

FISH IN BANANA-LEAF CUPS with white fish, shrimp, red curry paste, ground peanuts, coconut milk, egg, fish sauce, Chinese cabbage, coconut cream, and red chili

FISH IN COCONUT SAUCE with fish, coconut milk, fish sauce, cilantro, galangal, chilies, shallots, lemon grass, onions, and pepper

FISH WITH CHILI SAUCE with flounder, red chilies, garlic, fish sauce, and palm sugar

Serving Size	Calories	Fat (g)	Sodium (mg)	Carbohydrate (g)	Cholesterol (mg)	Fiber (g)
¾ cup	388.0	31.1	371.1	6.6	66.6	.99
9 oz (about 2 pieces)	**1106.5**	**105.9**	460.1	12.5	163.5	0.13
⅔ cup	303.3	21.5	349.4	3.5	84.0	.04
⅔ cup	259.7	17	209.3	10.6	115.6	0.24
¾ cup	410.8	26.0	107.6	12.4	86.5	5.98
1 cup	428.7	30.7	303.7	8.6	101.3	.14
3 oz	451.6	**32.1**	256.6	22.7	189.7	1.24
5 oz	242.2	14.1	456.8	7.1	220.5	1.56
5 oz	293.5	21.6	229.9	4.1	30.9	0.12
6 oz	504.3	16.5	501.2	2.1	232.0	.05

THAI DISHES

FOOD NAME

FISH WITH CILANTRO AND GARLIC with fish, lime juice, palm sugar, green onion, green and red chilies, broiled in banana leaves

FISH WITH GALANGAL with white fish, red chilies, garlic, shallots, lemon grass, fish sauce, wrapped in banana leaves

FISH WITH LEMON GRASS sole with garlic, red chilies, shallots, lime juice, lemon grass, and fish sauce

FISH WITH MUSHROOM SAUCE fish deep-fried, with onion, ginger root, shiitake mushrooms, and green onion

FISH WITH TAMARIND AND GINGER with fish, onion, garlic, ginger, fish sauce, soy sauce and palm sugar

MUSSELS WITH BASIL with mussels, garlic, lemon grass, and fish sauce

SHRIMP IN YELLOW SAUCE with shrimp, red chilies, red onion, lemon grass, turmeric, coconut milk, basil, and lime juice

SHRIMP WITH GARLIC with ginger, fish sauce, and cilantro

SHRIMP WITH MUSHROOMS *Goong Pahd Woonsen* with shrimp, red chili, ginger, garlic, shallots, lemon grass, fish sauce, and basil

STEAMED CRAB with garlic, shallot, cilantro, crabmeat, pork, egg, coconut cream, and fish sauce

STIR-FRIED SHRIMP AND GINGER with garlic, shallots, lime, fish sauce and green onions

THAI SEAFOOD DIP *Nam Prik* dried shrimp, fish sauce, garlic, chilies, and lime juice

Serving Size	Calories	Fat (g)	Sodium (mg)	Carbohydrate (g)	Cholesterol (mg)	Fiber (g)
1 6-oz fillet	273.5	11.3	90.4	5.8	98.0	.12
6 oz	148.7	3.0	319.3	1.8	41.1	.09
6 oz	543.3	18.9	648.1	7.6	232.0	.20
8 oz	**914.7**	46.9	**914.7**	22.1	232.0	1.02
6 oz	433.5	22.4	685.1	4.2	123.3	.23
10 mussels	489.9	12.2	**1411.1**	26.9	153.6	.04
4 large (1-oz) shrimp	191.2	8.5	242.6	5.9	162.5	0.09
4 large (1-oz) shrimp	185.1	8.8	305.1	3.7	162.5	.33
5 large (1-oz) shrimp	164.8	2.6	465.0	3.8	222.9	.31
3 oz	146.4	7.9	538.8	1.3	111.3	.06
4 large (1-oz) shrimp	210.3	9.9	346.5	4.3	185.7	.26
2 tblsp	16.2	0.2	141.7	1.0	18.6	.02

THAI DISHES

FOOD NAME

Desserts
Lowest Fat: Mango with Sticky Rice—9.9 g fat, 420.9 calories
Highest Fat: Coconut Custard—22.6 g fat, 315 calories

COCONUT CREPES   shredded coconut, rice flour, eggs, and coconut milk

COCONUT CUSTARD   eggs, coconut milk and sugar, topped with toasted almonds

MANGO WITH STICKY RICE   mango with sticky rice and coconut-cream sauce

Serving Size	Calories	Fat (g)	Sodium (mg)	Carbohydrate (g)	Cholesterol (mg)	Fiber (g)
1 crepe	240.4	15.7	57.8	23.2	54.8	1.77
¾ cup	315	22.6	94.3	22.6	340.0	0.63
10 oz	420.9	9.9	154.1	79.8	0.0	0.88

Staples

Ethnic foods include familiar staples such as breads, cheeses, fruits, nuts, vegetables, rice, noodles, common snacks and meat and egg dishes that are part of our everyday diet. Use these listings of basic foods to calculate the nutritional counts of dishes not listed elsewhere in this book.

STAPLES

FOOD NAME

Breads

- BAGEL
- KAISER ROLL
- FRENCH BREAD
- PITA BREAD
- PUMPERNICKEL
- RAISIN BREAD
- RYE
- SEVEN-GRAIN
- SOURDOUGH
- WHEAT
- WHITE

Dairy and Eggs

- BUTTER, SALTED
- BUTTER, UNSALTED

Cheeses

- CHEDDAR
- COTTAGE
- CREAM
- FETA
- GOAT'S MILK
- MONTEREY, JACK

Serving Size	Calories	Fat (g)	Sodium (mg)	Carbohydrate (g)	Cholesterol (mg)	Fiber (g)
1 bagel	240	0.8	170	47	0	0.2
1 roll	170	2.8	328	32.4	7	2
1 1-oz slice	65	0.9	136	12.1	0	0.4
½ 8-inch bread	330	4.2	534.5	62.8	0	0.2
1 1-oz slice	70	0.7	182	12.6	0	1
1 1-oz slice	62	1.3	107	12.4	0	0.9
1 1-oz slice	70	1	150	14.6	0	0.7
1 1-oz slice	90	1	170	16.6	0	0.8
1 slice	70	1	140	12.5	0	0.7
1 slice	60	1.5	120	11	0	1.4
1 1-oz slice	62	0.8	117	11.6	0	0
1 tblsp	101	11.5	117	0	31	0
1 tblsp	101	11.5	1	0	31	0
2 oz	228	18.8	352	6	60	0
2 oz	60	2.6	230	1.8	8	0
2 oz	198	19.8	168	1.5	62	0
2 oz	150	12	632	2.3	50	0
2 oz	164	13.6	360	1.8	40	0
2 oz	212	17.8	302	0.4	52	0

STAPLES

FOOD NAME

PARMESAN
RICOTTA
SWISS
CREAM, LIGHT
CREAM, HALF-AND-HALF
CREAM, HEAVY
CREAM, WHIPPED
CREAM, SOUR
EGG, WHOLE
EGG WHITE
EGG YOLK
ICE CREAM, CHOCOLATE
ICE CREAM, VANILLA
MAYONNAISE
MILK, WHOLE
MILK, 2%
MILK, SKIM
Fruits and Nuts
APPLE
APPLESAUCE (SWEETENED)
APPLESAUCE (UNSWEETENED)
APRICOT
AVOCADO

Serving Size	Calories	Fat (g)	Sodium (mg)	Carbohydrate (g)	Cholesterol (mg)	Fiber (g)
2 oz	257.5	17	1053.3	2.1	44.1	0
½ cup	214	16	103.5	3.7	62	0
2 oz	214	14.4	158	2	52	0
2 tblsp	55.1	5.5	11.1	1	19	0
2 tblsp	37	3.3	12	1.2	10	0
2 tblsp	98	10.5	11.1	0.8	39	0
2 tblsp	52	5.6	6	0.4	21	0
2 tblsp	61.6	6	15.4	1.2	12.8	0
1 large	79	5	63	0.6	213	0
1 large	16	0	55	0.4	0	0
1 large	63	5.6	8	0	213	0
½ cup	180	16	65	18	30	0
½ cup	175	11.8	54	16	44	0
1 tblsp	99	11	78.4	0.4	5	0
½ cup	75	4.1	60	5.7	16.5	0
½ cup	60	2.5	61	6	9	0
½ cup	43	0.2	63	6	2	0
5 oz	81	0.5	1	21	0	1.1
½ cup	152.5	0.5	10	25	0	1.5
½ cup	105	0.5	5	14	0	1.5
6 oz	76.5	0.6	1.5	17.6	0	1
6 oz	324	30.8	21	14.8	0	4.2

STAPLES

FOOD NAME
BANANA
BLUEBERRIES
CANTALOUPE
CASHEWS (DRY ROASTED, UNSALTED)
CHERRIES
CHESTNUTS
DATES
GRAPES (GREEN)
GRAPEFRUIT
MANGO
ORANGE
PEACH
PEANUTS (SALTED, OIL-ROASTED)
PEANUTS (UNSALTED, DRY-ROASTED)
PEAR (BARTLETT)
PECANS (DRY ROASTED, UNSALTED)
PINE NUTS (DRY-ROASTED, UNSALTED)
PINEAPPLE
PISTACHIOS (DRIED, UNSALTED)
PLANTAINS (COOKED)

Serving Size	Calories	Fat (g)	Sodium (mg)	Carbohydrate (g)	Cholesterol (mg)	Fiber (g)
5 oz	85.1	0.4	0.8	21.6	0	0.5
½ cup	41	0.3	4.5	10.3	0	0.9
8 oz	95	0.1	24.5	23.8	0	2.1
½ cup shelled	**392.5**	**32**	10.5	20.5	0	0.9
½ cup	52	0.7	0.5	12	0	0.3
½ cup (6 whole chestnuts)	155	1.4	5	33.7	0	0.8
2 oz (10 pitted dates)	228	0.4	2	61	0	1.8
3 oz (20 grapes)	70	0.1	.01	18.4	0	0.4
8 oz (½ large grapefruit)	42	0.1	0	11.4	0	0.4
1 10-oz mango	135	0.6	4	35	0	1.7
1 6-oz orange	62	0.2	0	15.4	0	0.6
1 4-oz peach	37	0.1	0	9.7	0	0.6
½ cup shelled	**419**	**35.5**	312.5	13.6	0	1.9
½ cup shelled	**428**	**36.3**	4.5	15.9	0	1.9
1 6-oz pear	98	0.7	1	25	0	2.3
½ cup shelled	355.3	35	2.3	13.1	0	0.7
½ cup shelled	406.8	32.3	2.3	13.1	0	0.7
1 cup	77	0.7	1	19.2	9	0.8
½ cup shelled	369.5	31	3.5	15.9	0	1.2
5 oz	90.5	0.3	3	23.6	0	0.4

STAPLES

FOOD NAME
PLUM
RAISINS (BLACK)
RAISINS (GOLDEN)
RASPBERRIES
SESAME SEEDS
STRAWBERRIES
WALNUTS
WATERMELON
Meat
BACON
CHICKEN (WHITE MEAT, SKINLESS)
CHICKEN (WHITE MEAT, WITH SKIN)
CHICKEN (DARK MEAT, WITH SKIN)
CHICKEN STOCK   with onions, celery, carrots, thyme, and parsley
CHORIZO SAUSAGE
CORNISH HEN
DUCK (WITH SKIN)
DUCK (WITHOUT SKIN)
GROUND BEEF, 30% Fat
GROUND BEEF, LEAN
HAM (ROASTED)

Serving Size	Calories	Fat (g)	Sodium (mg)	Carbohydrate (g)	Cholesterol (mg)	Fiber (g)
2 ½ oz	36	0.4	0	8.6	0	0.4
½ cup	214	0.4	21	56.9	0	0.9
½ cup	219	0.3	9	57.7	0	1
½ cup	31	0.3	0	7.1	0	1.8
1 tblsp	55	5	3.7	1.7	0	0.2
1 cup	45	0.6	2	10.4	0	0.8
½ cup shelled	325.5	32	1	7.9	0	1
½ cup diced	25	0	2	5.7	0	0.3
2 strips, fried	73.2	6.3	202.6	0.1	10.7	0
4 oz (½ breast)	188.9	4.1	85.1	0	97.1	0
4 oz (½ breast)	250	13.4	91	0	92	0
4 oz (2 small wings)	298.5	21.5	106.5	0	118.5	0
1 cup	39	0.9	776	0.9	1	0
1 oz	125	10.9	105	0	20	0
8 oz (1 hen)	300.6	8.2	85.1	0	149	0
8 oz (1 duck)	**927.2**	**90.4**	144.8	0	174.4	0
8 oz	**456.2**	25.4	148	0	202	0
4 oz	351	**30**	77	0	96	0
4 oz	306	21.3	86.6	0	98	0
4 oz	174.8	6.6	**1503.5**	0	64.8	0

STAPLES

FOOD NAME

- LAMB CHOP (BROILED)
- LAMB (LEG, FAT TRIMMED)
- LAMB, RACK OF
- LIVER (FRIED)
- PORK CHOP (BROILED)
- PORK CUTLET (BROILED)
- PORK, GROUND
- PRIME RIB
- SIRLOIN
- TENDERLOIN (FAT TRIMMED)
- TURKEY (LIGHT MEAT, WITHOUT SKIN)
- TURKEY (LIGHT MEAT, WITH SKIN)
- TURKEY (DARK MEAT, WITH SKIN)
- VEAL (BROILED)
- VEAL CHOP
- VEAL CUTLET

Noodles and Rice

- CHOW MEIN NOODLES
- EGG NOODLES
- MACARONI, ENRICHED
- RAVIOLI, CHEESE

Serving Size	Calories	Fat (g)	Sodium (mg)	Carbohydrate (g)	Cholesterol (mg)	Fiber (g)
1 4-oz shoulder chop	317.6	26.7	87.3	0	109.1	0
4 oz	231	10.4	81	0	104	0
4 oz (2 medium chops)	357.3	26.1	87.1	0	113.7	0
4 oz	246.6	9.3	120	0	546.6	0
1 4-oz chop	26.5	12.9	16.3	0	113.8	0
4 oz	291	17.3	85	0	108	0
4 oz	253	18.7	53.3	0	111	0
8 oz, cooked	**572.5**	**33**	167	0	186.2	0
8 oz, cooked	**610**	**38**	140	0	204	0
8 oz, cooked	481.1	24.6	144	0	192	0
4 oz	178.8	3.7	73	0	78	0
4 oz	223	9.4	71	0	86.2	0
4 oz	178.8	10.3	80.4	0	80.1	0
4 oz	185.3	9.3	56.3	0	109.5	0
4 oz	259	15.8	104.2	0	125.5	0
4 oz	230.3	5.8	76.3	0	159	0
1 cup cooked	237	13.8	197	25.9	0	1.8
1 cup cooked	212	2.4	11	37.3	50	0.2
1 cup cooked	151	1	1	32.2	0	0.1
1 cup cooked	360	8	220	1.5	65	0

STAPLES

FOOD NAME
RICE, BROWN
RICE, WHITE
PASTA, DRIED COMMERCIAL
Seafood
CLAMS
COD
CRAB
FISH ROE
FLOUNDER
HALIBUT
MONKFISH
OCTOPUS
SALMON
SEA BASS
SNAPPER
SOLE
SQUID
SWORDFISH
TUNA
Vegetables
ARTICHOKE (STEAMED)
ASPARAGUS (STEAMED)

Serving Size	Calories	Fat (g)	Sodium (mg)	Carbohydrate (g)	Cholesterol (mg)	Fiber (g)
1 cup cooked	352	1.8	8	76	0	0.8
1 cup cooked	354	0.8	5	78.5	0	0.2
1 cup cooked	155	0.6	1	32.2	0	0.2
3 oz	65.5	0.1	102	2.3	42.5	0
8 oz	186.2	1.5	122.4	0	98.4	0
2 oz	46.9	0.3	469.3	0	23.1	0
2 tblsp	80	5.8	480	1.2	188	0
8 oz	207.5	2.7	183.5	0	109.1	0
8 oz	247.4	5.2	122.4	0	71.8	0
8 oz	172.9	3.5	39.9	0	55.9	0
3 oz	69	0.9	691.6	1.8	42.1	0
8 oz	321.9	14.3	98.4	0	125	0
8 oz	216.2	20.8	128.1	0	96.3	0
8 oz	226.1	3	143.6	0	82.5	0
8 oz	206.3	3.5	186.7	0	154.3	0
3 oz	149	6.4	260	6.6	221	0
8 oz	274	9.1	202.2	0	87.8	0
8 oz	415	14.1	114.4	0	111.7	0
1 medium artichoke	61.3	0	114	13.3	0	1.3
4 oz (5 stalks)	30	0.3	2	4.9	0	1.1

STAPLES

FOOD NAME

BEANS, BLACK
BEANS, GREEN (STEAMED)
BEANS, LIMA
BEANS, PINTO
BEAN SPROUTS
BEETS
BLACK-EYED PEAS
BROCCOLI
BRUSSELS SPROUTS
CABBAGE, BOK CHOY
CABBAGE, GREEN
CABBAGE, RED
CARROTS
CAULIFLOWER
CHICKPEAS
COLLARDS
CORN
EGGPLANT
LENTILS
PEAS, GREEN
PEAS, SNOW

Serving Size	Calories	Fat (g)	Sodium (mg)	Carbohydrate (g)	Cholesterol (mg)	Fiber (g)
½ cup cooked	339	1.5	25	61	0	0
½ cup	20.4	0	3.6	4.7	0	0.7
½ cup cooked	104	0.3	14.5	20	0	1.8
½ cup cooked	331.5	1.2	9.5	60.5	0	4
½ cup cooked	15	0.3	5	3.9	0	0.8
½ cup cooked	30	0.1	49	6.8	0	0.5
½ cup cooked	89	0.7	1	15	0	0
½ cup cooked	24	0.3	24	4.6	0	0.9
6 oz cooked (about 8 sprouts)	76	0.5	44	15.8	0	2.6
½ cup cooked	10	0.1	30.2	1.4	0	1.38
½ cup cooked	16	0.1	14.2	3.6	0	0.5
½ cup cooked	16	0.1	6.2	3.6	0	1.8
4 oz cooked	51	0.2	75	11.9	0	2.2
1 cup cooked	24	0.2	7	4.9	0	2.5
½ cup cooked	134	2.1	6	22.5	0	2.9
½ cup cooked	17	0.1	16	3	0	0.4
½ cup cooked	89	20.6	14	20.6	0	1
1 cup cooked	22	0.1	2	5	0	0.8
½ cup cooked	106	0	0	19.3	0	1.2
½ cup cooked	65	0.3	3.5	12.5	0	1.6
½ cup cooked	34	0.2	3.5	5.6	0	1.9

STAPLES

FOOD NAME

- PICKLE, DILL
- PICKLE, SWEET
- POTATO, BAKED IN SKIN
- POTATO, FRIED IN OIL
- PUMPKIN
- RUTABAGA
- SPINACH
- SWEET POTATO (BAKED)
- TOMATO
- ZUCCHINI

Sweets

- CARAMEL
- MARASCHINO CHERRIES
- CHOCOLATE, MILK
- CHOCOLATE, DARK
- CHOCOLATE FUDGE SAUCE
- JAMS, JELLIES, PRESERVES
- MARSHMALLOWS
- SUGAR, BROWN
- SUGAR, GRANULATED
- SYRUP, CORN
- SYRUP, MAPLE

Serving Size	Calories	Fat (g)	Sodium (mg)	Carbohydrate (g)	Cholesterol (mg)	Fiber (g)
5 oz	16	0.1	400.5	2.9	0	0.4
1 2½-inch pickle	20	0.2	107	5.1	0	0.3
4 oz	124	0.1	9	28.6	0	0.7
2 oz	315	21.1	282	30.6	0	1.1
1½ cups raw	8.2	0	0.5	2	0	0.3
3 oz raw	32.5	0.1	3.5	7.7	0	0.7
½ cup cooked	21	0.2	63.5	3.4	0	0.5
5 oz	136	0.4	17	32	0	1
1 5-oz tomato	30	0.3	12.5	6.6	0	0.7
4 oz cooked	18.1	0.1	3.3	4	0	0.6
1 oz	115	3	64	23	1	0
1 cherry	16.5	0.1	2.5	4.2	0	0.1
1 oz	145	9	23	16	6	0.1
1 oz	140	9	1	17	0	0.3
2 tblsp	125	5	41	21	0	0.1
2 tblsp	108	0	4	28	0	0.2
1 oz	100	0	25	25	0	0
1 tblsp	51.7	0	4.2	13.4	0	0
1 tblsp	46	0	0	11.9	0	0
2 tblsp	120	0	60	30	0	0
2 tblsp	100	0	4	25	0	0

Weekly Food Chart

WEEKLY FOOD CHART

234

MONDAY	Food
Breakfast	
Lunch	
Dinner	
Monday Totals	

Serving Size	Calories	Fat (g)	Sodium (mg)	Carbohydrate (g)	Cholesterol (mg)	Fiber (g)

WEEKLY FOOD CHART

236

TUESDAY	Food
Breakfast	
Lunch	
Dinner	
Tuesday Totals	

Serving Size	Calories	Fat (g)	Sodium (mg)	Carbohydrate (g)	Cholesterol (mg)	Fiber (g)

WEEKLY FOOD CHART

238

WEDNESDAY	Food
Breakfast	
Lunch	
Dinner	
Wednesday Totals	

Serving Size	Calories	Fat (g)	Sodium (mg)	Carbohydrate (g)	Cholesterol (mg)	Fiber (g)

WEEKLY FOOD CHART

240

THURSDAY	Food
Breakfast	
Lunch	
Dinner	
Thursday Totals	

Serving Size	Calories	Fat (g)	Sodium (mg)	Carbohydrate (g)	Cholesterol (mg)	Fiber (g)

WEEKLY FOOD CHART

242

FRIDAY	Food
Breakfast	
Lunch	
Dinner	
Friday Totals	

Serving Size	Calories	Fat (g)	Sodium (mg)	Carbohydrate (g)	Cholesterol (mg)	Fiber (g)

WEEKLY FOOD CHART

244

SATURDAY	Food
Breakfast	
Lunch	
Dinner	
Saturday Totals	

	Serving Size	Calories	Fat (g)	Sodium (mg)	Carbohydrate (g)	Cholesterol (mg)	Fiber (g)

WEEKLY FOOD CHART

SUNDAY	Food
Breakfast	
Lunch	
Dinner	
Sunday Totals	

	Serving Size	Calories	Fat (g)	Sodium (mg)	Carbohydrate (g)	Cholesterol (mg)	Fiber (g)

WEEKLY FOOD CHART

248

DAILY TOTALS	
Monday	
Tuesday	
Wednesday	
Thursday	
Friday	
Saturday	
Sunday	
WEEKLY TOTALS	

Serving Size	Calories	Fat (g)	Sodium (mg)	Carbohydrate (g)	Cholesterol (mg)	Fiber (g)